THE **CRUNCH** FITNESS GUIDES

PERFECT POSTURE

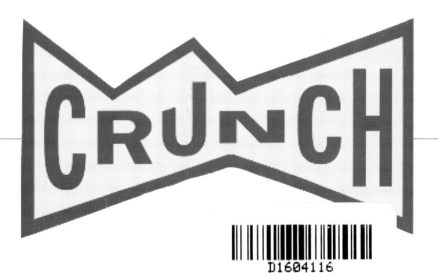

D1604116

HATHERLEIGH

NEW YORK

Getfitnow.com Books
An Independent Imprint of Hatherleigh Press

Getfitnow.com Books
An Independent Imprint of Hatherleigh Press
an affiliate of W.W. Norton & Company
500 Fifth Avenue
New York, NY 10110
1-800-367-2550
www.getfitnow.com

Before beginning any strenuous exercise program consult your physician. The author and publisher of this book and workout disclaim any liability, personal or professional, resulting from the misapplication of any of the training procedures described in this publication.

Library of Congress Cataloging in-Publication Data

Perfect posture / Crunch.
     p.cm. -- (The Crunch fitness series)
   ISBN 1-57826-040-X
   1. Posture. 2. Stretching exercises. I. Crunch. II. Series.

RA781.5 .P47 2000
613. 7'8--dc21

                                                                    99-087620

Series Editor: Heather Ogilvie
Cover design: Lisa Fyfe
Text design and composition: John Reinhardt Book Design
Photographs: Chia Messina

Printed in Canada on acid-free paper

10   9   8   7   6   5   4   3   2   1

MVFOl

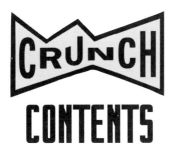

CONTENTS

PART 1

Your Mother Was Right
(or The Importance of Good Posture)

PART 2

Assessing Your Posture

PART 3

How Exercise Can Improve Your Posture

PART 4

The Stable Spine

PART 5

The Upper Body Workout

PART 6

The Lower Body Workout

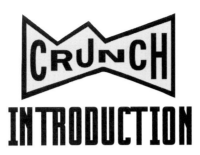

INTRODUCTION

Welcome to CRUNCH! For over a decade, we've been welcoming people of all shapes, sizes, ages, and fitness levels to our gyms. As we've expanded from a tiny, one-room aerobics studio in New York's East Village to cities across the country (and even to Tokyo), we've offered group fitness classes, personal training, and equipment to appeal to everyone from stressed-out workaholics and jet setters to senior citizens and expectant moms. We're living up to our motto, "No Judgements!"

We're aware that some people shy away from joining a gym or from starting a fitness program because they think it demands too great a change in their lifestyle. But at CRUNCH, we believe you shouldn't have to change your lifestyle in order to be fit. In fact, we believe your workout should change to fit your lifestyle. It is our firm belief that the success of a fitness program has nothing to do with how many hours you spend in the gym, but how good you feel when you're outside the gym, living your life.

That's why we've created these guides—to show you that no matter what your lifestyle, there's a workout you can do that will complement it and get you fit. For example, we designed the *Road Warrior Workout* for people who spend a lot of time traveling on business. These folks don't have to give up their fitness programs—in fact, by doing a workout specially adapted to life on the road, they can maintain their fitness level and become less susceptible to all the common aches and discomforts of travel.

Get Fit in a CRUNCH is for those people who are trying to shape up in time for a big event—a wedding, a reunion, a trip to the beach. Based on CRUNCH's popular class, Emergency Beach Training, *Get Fit in a CRUNCH* lays out a safe, effective four-week workout, 12-week workout, and six-month workout.

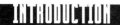

Since the hardest part of any fitness program is starting it, we've written *Beginner's Luck* to help people stay motivated and become more familiar with—and less intimidated by—basic cardiovascular and strength training exercises. It's a workout you can take at your own pace, according to your own goals.

Other CRUNCH guides include *The Workaholic's Workout*, targeting time-pressed workaholics; *On Your Mark. Get Set. Go! Marathon Training*, for first-time marathon runners; and *Posture Perfect*, for people who want to eliminate or avoid common back pain and improve posture.

At CRUNCH, we don't want you to conform to some workout fad or a lifestyle of spending more time at the gym than at play. We want to give you workout options that will conform to your lifestyle—without judgement.

Doug Levine
Founder and CEO
Crunch Fitness International, Inc.
www.crunch.com

ABOUT THE AUTHOR

Dr. Scott G. Duke designed the workouts in *Perfect Posture*. The President of Duke Chiropractic, P.C., in New York City, Dr. Duke is a board-certified chiropractic sports physician. He has extensive experience in the treatment of competitive athletes, assisting them in optimizing their physical performance levels. Dr. Duke has served as Sports Chiropractor at the United States Olympic Training Center, as well as at the United States Competitive and World Aerobics Championships. In addition to consulting for Crunch, he also consults for American Fitness Center (N.Y.), New York Sports Club, Sutton Gymnastics, and the United Nations Athletic Club (N.Y.), and he is the Advisory Board Sports Physician for Equinox Fitness Center (N.Y.).

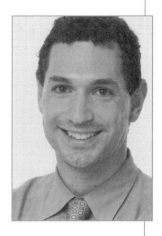

Dr. Duke is certified by the American Board of Chiropractic Sports Physicians as a Diplomate in Sports Injuries; a Medical Exercise Specialist by the American Academy of Health and Fitness Professionals; the National Strength and Conditioning Association as a strength and conditioning specialist; and by the American College of Sports Medicine in Health and Fitness.

Dr. Duke was past strength and conditioning coach for the Chicago Blackhawks professional hockey team. In addition to making appearances on FOX 5 *Good Day New York*, Dr. Duke has published and lectured throughout the United States and Canada on topics of sports performance enhancement techniques, athletic injury, rehabilitation, spinal stabilization, and flexibility.

A faculty member of the American Council of Exercise, Dr. Duke educates the personal training community to assist in the reduction of injuries in the health club setting. His protocol for exercise prescription has been adopted by Elite Health Club facilities in New York City.

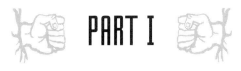

PART I

YOUR MOTHER WAS RIGHT

(OR, THE IMPORTANCE OF GOOD POSTURE)

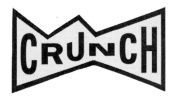

Remember your mother's stern commands? "Get your elbows off the table!" "Don't talk with your mouth full!" "Sit up straight!" As kids, we questioned the importance of such edicts on a daily basis. What was the big deal about how you sat or stood, anyway? Time was, posture was something only beauty pageant contestants needed to learn—by walking with books on their heads.

Now, as you sink deeper into the couch, as your shoulders hunch over your computer, as you start to think you may actually be shrinking—well, all of a sudden, posture has become a big deal.

Posture is how you "hold yourself" or "carry yourself." If you stand tall, with your shoulders back, chest high, and back straight, you're on your way to good posture. If your shoulders are rounded, your neck falls forward, and your head droops, you have poor posture. Your body language conveys sadness, weakness, shyness, and resignation. What's more, the more "hunched over" you become, the harder it is to straighten yourself out because your spine becomes fused in the position.

Why is good posture so difficult to maintain? First of all, if you have bad posture habits, you must make a constant, conscious effort to hold yourself differently—and that means using muscles you haven't used in a while. What's more, many people who are attempting to achieve good posture overcompensate for the rounding forward effect. They throw their shoulders too far back and arch their backs in an unhealthy way. This posture does more harm than good.

Even people who think they have generally good posture find out—from suffering back injuries while doing everyday activities—that their back muscles are not as strong as they thought they were and that their posture could use improvement. People active in sports or who regularly work out in gyms—people who may be in great overall shape and good health—can actually be among the most vulnerable to common back pain and spine injuries. While they may occasionally ask themselves, "Am I sitting up straight at my desk?" or "Is my mattress giving me the proper support?" they probably never ask themselves, "Is my spine stable and in the correct position to lift this dumbbell or do this lat pull-down?" How you position your spine while exercising is just as important as how you position your spine while resting.

THE CONSEQUENCES OF POOR POSTURE

Obviously, poor posture contributes to chronic back pain. But back pain is not all your mother was trying to spare you. Over time, poor posture can lead to premature degenerative disorders, such as herniated disks, sciatica, bowel/bladder discomfort, colitis, constipation, acid reflux disease, and nerve damage. Problems associated with poor upper back posture include scoliosis (rounding of the shoulders and upper back, with a resultant lateral shift to the spine), lung compression (which leads to breathing difficulties), and headaches. In fact, poor posture triggers migraines more often than certain foods do.

THE CAUSES OF COMMON BACK PAIN

Most people develop poor posture and chronic back pain when they sit for long periods of time—slouching in the classroom, slumping on the couch, hunching over a computer at their desks. Sitting without proper support is especially hard on your lower back.

Consider this: When you are lying on your back, your weight is evenly distributed over the length of your body. When you stand straight up, you put twice that weight (or all the weight of your upper body) on your lower back. But when you are sitting without back support, your lower back bears *three times* the amount of weight it did when you were lying down! That's because when you're standing, your legs help to support your upper body weight, but when you're sitting, all that weight comes down on your lower back. What's more, when you're driving, your lower back bears *three to five times* the weight, depending on the amount of shock absorption your back must endure (in this regard, SUVs are much worse than sedans).

In addition to sitting with poor or no back support, some other causes of common back pain are:

- Wearing ill-fitting shoes and high heels.
- Lying on an uneven mattress with inadequate back support.
- Crossing your legs while sitting.
- Experiencing emotional stress.
- Running on the same surface and in the same direction (e.g., with or against traffic) day after day.
- Running without stretching. This often causes "runner's knee," also known as the IT band syndrome. The iliotibial (IT) band, the tissue that surrounds the outer leg, becomes overdeveloped and performs hip abduction, which the hip abductor muscles should, and would, perform if they were properly stretched. The symptom of IT band syndrome is pain on the outer sides of the kneecap. Proper stretching can reverse the effects of the syndrome.
- Working out with weights without stretching properly.
- Working one muscle group till it is far more developed than its counterpart muscle group, which is usually weak and vulnerable to pulls and tears. Such muscle imbalances lead to serious back injuries as well as contributing to poor posture. (People often work their front muscles, such as their biceps, chest, and quads, far more than they work their back muscles, such as their triceps, middle traps, glutes, and hamstrings.)
- Doing yoga without first achieving spinal stabilization and proper flexibility.

Among physically active people, one of the leading causes of back pain is failing to stretch out the proper muscles before exercising. And, at the gym, people tend to just start exercising on whatever equipment happens to be available at the time, instead of giving some thought to the order in which they should do their exercises. For example, attempting to lift a weight with one muscle before its opposite (and supporting) muscle has been warmed up could lead to a back injury. Fatiguing the small muscle groups (such as forearms and calves) before the large muscle groups (such as hamstrings and glutes) can also lead to injury. Trainers refer to this practice as the improper sequencing of exercises. *You should always exercise large muscle groups before small ones.*

Improving posture by correcting the problems described above can help you avoid back pain and common back injuries. The exercises we describe later in the book can help you stretch and strengthen the muscles that are responsible for maintaining good posture. But first, let's see just how susceptible you are to typical posture problems.

PART II
ASSESSING YOUR POSTURE

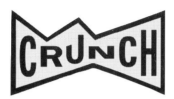

You can analyze your posture from two perspectives: static and dynamic. When you are not moving—for example, when you're lying down, sitting, or standing—your posture is said to be "static." When you are moving, your posture is "dynamic."

Look at the examples of good and bad static posture on the following page. Stand in front of a mirror. Does your posture have similar features to those in the photos shown?

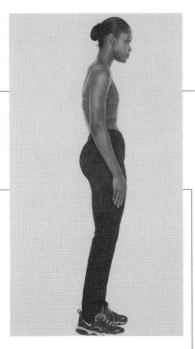

Static Posture

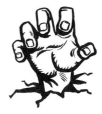

Here, notice how the shoulders are rounded, the upper back is hunched, the neck juts forward, and the head droops. This posture is very common, and, if nothing is done to correct it, this woman will become more and more hunched over as she ages.

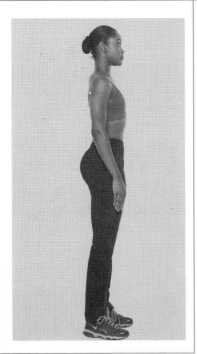

Now the woman is demonstrating good standing posture. Her shoulders are back, chest expanded, neck straight, and head high, lined up with her shoulders (from a side view). Notice that she has no pronounced arch or sway in her lower back (a slight arch may be perfectly normal). That's because she is standing with what's called a "pelvic tilt" or "neutral spine position."

Here's how to do a pelvic tilt: When you stand, think about "flattening" your lower back, so that if you were standing up against a wall, your lower back would be parallel to it. This motion requires you to contract your abdominal muscles slightly in order to "tilt" your pelvis back. However, too flat of a lower back curve is just as bad as too much of a lower back curve. "Neutral spine" is the position in between that feels natural for your physique.

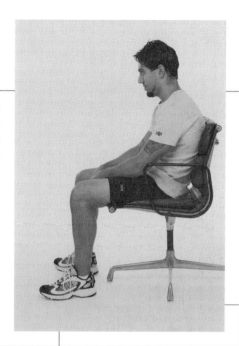

Here, notice how the person's lower back and shoulders are rounded. This common posture feels as though you've "sunk" into your chair. Most people end up in this position by the end of the workday. If you find yourself in this position from the get-go, then you can bet your supportive posture muscles are not balanced and are probably weak, tight, and vulnerable to injury, especially if you exercise in a health club setting.

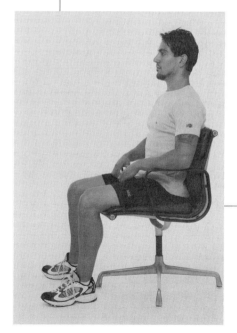

This man is now demonstrating good sitting posture. Notice how his butt is all the way back, touching the back of the chair. His lower back is also touching the seat back, giving him good support. His shoulders are back and his feet are flat on the floor. His back demonstrates a natural curve (called "lordosis") to the spine.

REST EASY

You can achieve good posture while sleeping in several ways. The easiest is to lie on your side with your knees bent up toward your chest (like the fetal position), and with a pillow between your knees and another under your neck and head. The pillow helps to take pressure off your hips, especially if you're a woman. Another position is to lie on your back with a blanket or small pillow under your knees and another under the curve of your neck. Lying on your stomach, however, can cause your lower back to arch and is not recommended for most people. If you must lie on your stomach, due to years of bad habits, try placing a flat cushion under your pelvis to reduce the sway in your lower back.

DYNAMIC POSTURE

The Lunge Test. To assess your dynamic posture, take the lunge test. Standing straight, with your hands on your hips, lunge to a full stride in front of you.

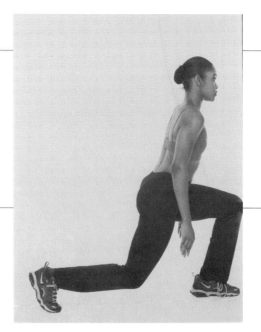

Does your torso drift forward during the lunge, as shown here? If so, you probably have tight hip flexors and weak gluteal muscles. (We'll discuss more about these muscles in Chapter 3.)

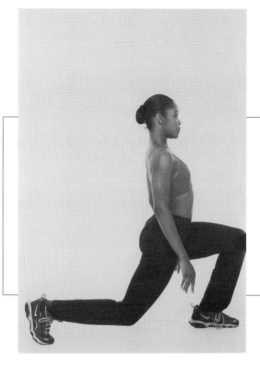

Do you have increased "hyperlordosis," or an arched back, during the lunge, as in this photo? If so, you probably have tight spinal erectors (spine muscles) and weak abdominals as well.

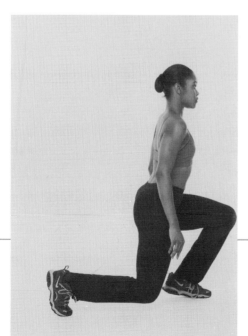

Does your front leg's heel lift off the floor, as shown here? If so, your calf muscles are tight.

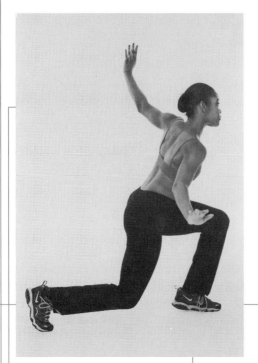

Does your front knee shake during the lunge? If so, your quadriceps are weak and you may have balance ("proprioception") problems. You could possibly have instability in your knee or your ankle (due to loss of structural integrity to the cartilage or ligaments).

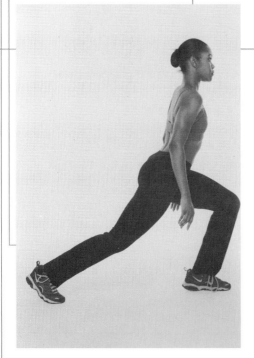

Does your front knee go past your front toe? Your stride may be too short due to tight hamstrings. Do you have difficulty placing your back knee to the ground (i.e., do you feel a pull on your rear leg's kneecap)? If so, your back leg hip flexors and quads are too tight. People who do lunges using this form are prone to kneecap injuries.

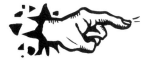

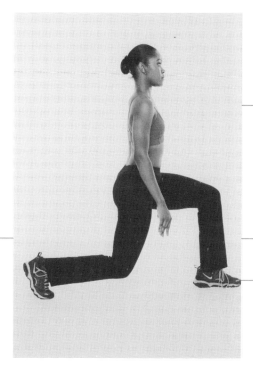

Here's a lunge with good form! Notice how the front knee is in line with the front heel and the upright torso is vertically aligned.

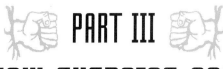

PART III
HOW EXERCISE CAN IMPROVE YOUR POSTURE

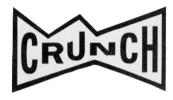

Improving your posture is not as simple as remembering to sit up straight at the dinner table. You must develop strong *and* flexible neck and back muscles. This means stretching tight muscles and strengthening weak ones.

As described in the previous chapters, most back pain is caused by muscle imbalances: one muscle is highly developed, but its opposite muscle is weak and underdeveloped. For example, you may have strong abdominal muscles from doing crunches. These muscles run vertically and obliquely down the front of your torso. But if you haven't exercised their opposite muscles, the spinal erectors, which run down the length of your back and support your spine, those muscles could be especially weak, tight, and prone to injury. When one muscle (or muscle group) is extremely developed, the opposite muscles tend to become weak or especially tight. Another example is the hip flexor muscles, which tend to be overdeveloped (usually from doing crunches incorrectly) in comparison with their counterpart muscles, the gluteus maximus.

A muscle and its counterpart are also referred to as the "agonist" and its "antagonist." Tightness and overdevelopment in agonist muscles can lead to weakness in antagonist muscles, and vice versa. Technically, this condition is known as Sherington's law of reciprocal inhibition. For example, say your hip flexors become tight from overuse. This tightness will not only mechanically limit the motion of the antagonist muscles, the hip extensors, but it will neurologically inhibit and weaken the action of those muscles as well. This combination of biomechanics and neurophysiology creates and maintains muscle imbalances that lead to poor posture and eventual spinal injury.

Here's another way to look at Sherington's law: Because tight, over-developed agonist muscles weaken their antagonist muscles, *simply stretching tight muscles will neurologically strengthen the weak antagonist muscles—without doing strength training exercises!*

Here's a list of agonist and antagonist muscles. (We'll describe stretching or strengthening exercises for them later in the book.)

Agonist (Tight)	Antagonist (Weak)

NECK

SCM*, suboccipitals	deep neck flexors
upper trapezius, levator scapulae	lower trapezius

CHEST/SHOULDERS

anterior deltoids	posterior deltoids
pectoralis major/minor	rhomboids, middle trapezius
latissimus dorsi	serratus anterior

LOWER BACK

spinal erectors	abdominals, gluteus maximus
QLs*	gluteus medius

HIPS

hip flexors (psoas, rectus femoris)	abdominals, gluteus maximus
hip rotators (piriformis, TFL*)	gluteus medius
adductors	VMOs,* gluteus medius
hamstrings	gluteus maximus, quadriceps

*SCM is the sternocleidomastoid; QLs are the quadratus lumborum; TFL is the tensorfascialatae; and VMOs are the vastus medialis obliques (quad group), which, when weak, are a common cause of kneecap injuries.

Such muscle imbalances lead to two common posture problems: the Upper Crossed Syndrome and the Lower Crossed Syndrome.

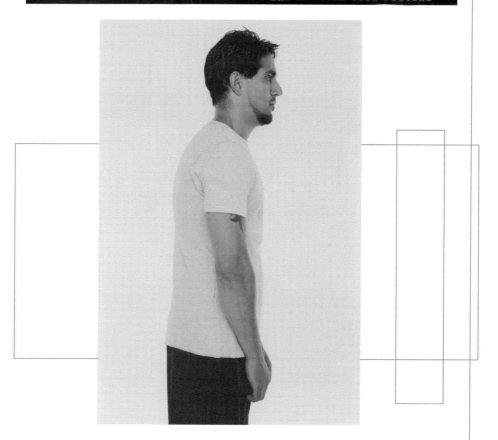

The Upper Crossed Syndrome

This condition affects the shape of your neck and upper back. Your upper back hunches, your shoulders round forward, your neck juts forward, and your head droops down.

In this syndrome, the muscles of your chest (pectorals and anterior delts), front and back of the neck (SCM, levator scapulae, suboccipitals), and upper back (upper traps and latissimus dorsi) are tight. The muscles of your middle back (rhomboids, middle and lower traps, rear delts, and serratus anterior) and your deep neck flexors are weak.

In other words, if the muscles of the back of your neck are tight, then the rest of your neck muscles are probably weak. If your chest feels tight, then the muscles of your upper back are weak. You cannot bring your neck and shoulders back, so they routinely slouch forward and further tighten, resulting in a pronounced head jut and rounded upper back.

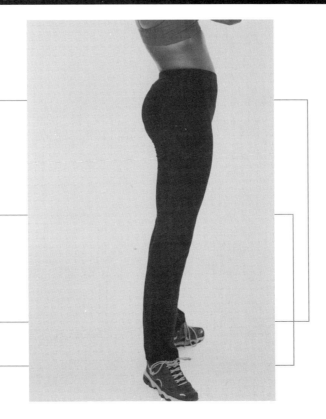

The Lower Crossed Syndrome

This condition is the culprit behind most lower back problems, where herniated disks and sciatica most often occur. The hip flexors, spinal erectors, TFL, piriformis, and QLs are tight and overdeveloped, while the gluteus maximus, gluteus medius, and abdominal muscles are weak. (The hamstrings and adductors are also usually tight.) In this syndrome, the abdomen may protrude, the lower back arches, and one or both feet turn out. This posture places a great amount of stress on the disks in the lower back. As the abs get relatively weak, the QLs and hip flexors tighten and further stress the lower portion of the spine—until a simple twist or forward bend "pulls your back out"!

Chapter 5 describes an upper body workout, including stretches and strengthening exercises, that will help you prevent or reverse the effects of the Upper Crossed Syndrome. Chapter 6 describes a lower body workout that will help you prevent or reverse the effects of the Lower Crossed Syndrome. As you do these workouts, however, it's essential that you maintain a stable spine. Chapter 4 will show you how to stabilize your spine and recognize good dynamic posture.

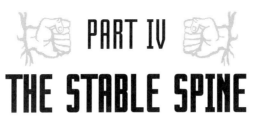

PART IV
THE STABLE SPINE

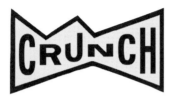

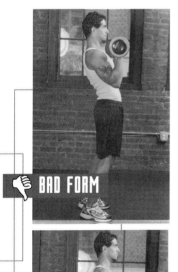

BAD FORM

GOOD FORM

The most important thing to do before working out, especially with weights, is to stabilize your spine. When you are lifting, pushing, or pulling a weight, you want to work only the intended muscle. Many people, however, unwittingly use their back to help them perform exercises intended for a different muscle group—for example, their biceps. Not only does this reduce the benefit to the bicep, but it can also lead to very serious back injuries.

straining your back, you should avoid weights that are too heavy and require momentum to complete the movement. To make sure you are not using momentum, which will bring your back muscles into play, you should find what is called "neutral spine position." When your spine is in this position, you place the least amount of tension and stress on your spinal muscles, joints, ligaments, and disks.

To find your neutral spine position, sit on a bench or a chair without any back support. Feel your upper body weight distributed evenly across your butt. Hold yourself erect, but do not push your shoulders too far back, thus arching your lower back. (Your lower back may have a natural sway to it, but you shouldn't encourage a pronounced sway.) Gently rock your pelvis forward and backward and from side to side until it feels comfortable. Slightly contract your abdominals. (Doing so achieves the neutral pelvic tilt described in Chapter 2.) Tense your core so that if you were to do a bicep curl, lifting a dumbbell from your hip to your chest, your back would not move. This is spinal stabilization.

This stable spine position, with natural lumbar curve, is the correct posture to assume when you are doing any strength training exercise. Even when your back is supported, as on a leg press machine, you can easily hurt your back if you are not maintaining a stable spine.

THE PHYSIOBALL NEUTRAL SPINE

Another, and easier, way to find neutral spine position is to use a physioball. Physioballs are available for general use at Crunch gyms and for sale at sporting goods stores. To choose the right size ball, sit

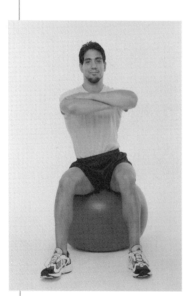

on the ball with your feet flat on the floor. Ninety-degree angles should form at your knees and hips. If the angles are lesser or greater than 90 degrees, try a larger or smaller ball.

To find your neutral spine position on the physioball, sit on the ball and bounce forward, backward, and from side to side. Rock your pelvis several times. Use this as a guide to explore which position feels most comfortable for your back. As you come to a stop, tighten your core muscles to lock your spine in this position. Your spine position should now be neutral for your physique. Your upper back should be fairly straight and your lower back should be slightly arched to contain the natural curve of your lower spine. If you slouch, the ball should start to roll out from under you. Neutral spine position gives you control of the ball.

To practice finding and maintaining neutral spine position throughout a complete range of motion, do the following 12 series of floor stabilization exercises. (The first seven series do not require a physioball.)

SPINAL STABILIZATION EXERCISES

Perform as many of the following 12 series of exercises as you can, once or twice a week, leaving at least one day of rest between exercise sessions. Each series of exercises is more difficult than the last, so don't expect to do all of them easily on the first day. Looks can be deceiving—these exercises are more difficult than they may look. *Do not move on to the next series until you can complete the first series with ease.* The first few series build the foundation for performing the more difficult series. Once you can complete all the series with relative ease, you are ready to move on to the workouts described in Chapters 5 and 6, which will help you maintain proper posture and help prevent degenerative spinal disease.

All the exercises here are intended for healthy readers. If you have any prior or existing back pain or if your neck or back begins to hurt as a result of the exercises, stop all exercises and have your back evaluated by a physician who understands spinal mechanics before you continue this exercise program.

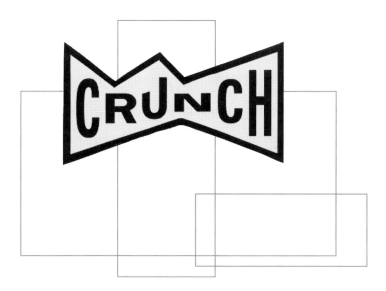

SERIES 1: ABDOMINAL BRACING

Difficulty performing the following pelvic tilts is a result of poor coordination and lack of mobility in the lower spine due to tight, overactive spinal erector muscles. (Chiropractic care may be a first line of defense to help minimize future lack of coordination and possible injury.)

Abdominal bracing is the primary concept with regard to performing all the subsequent progressive exercises in this chapter (as well as gym exercises in general). If you cannot master these different torso bracing positions, then do *not* move on, as injury may occur.

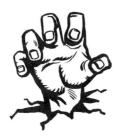

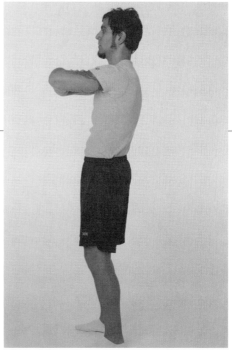

Standing ab bracing

Stand with your feet slightly apart, your knees slightly bent, and your arms crossed in front of you. Tilt your pelvis forward then backward into a posterior pelvic tilt. Brace your abs and hold the position for five seconds. Breathe out while holding the contraction. Repeat three times.

This exercise is excellent for people who are on their feet all day.

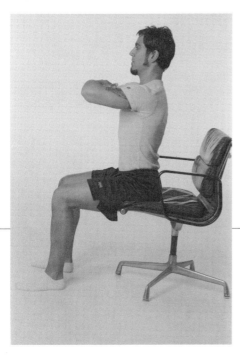

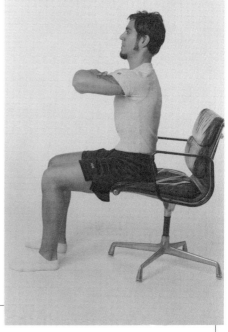

Seated ab bracing

Sit on the edge of a chair with your arms folded in front of you. Arch your back, then flatten your lower spine. This will help you find a neutral position that is comfortable. Hold the position for five seconds, while exhaling. Repeat three times, holding each rep for five seconds. This exercise is excellent for those who sit a great deal.

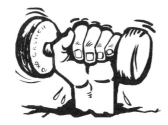

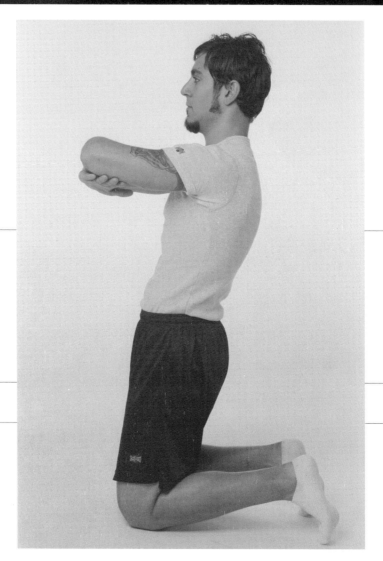

Kneeling ab bracing

Kneel on the floor with your arms crossed in front of you. Perform a posterior pelvic tilt, bracing your abs and contracting your glutes. Do three reps, holding each rep for five seconds. Remember to exhale while you're holding the contraction.

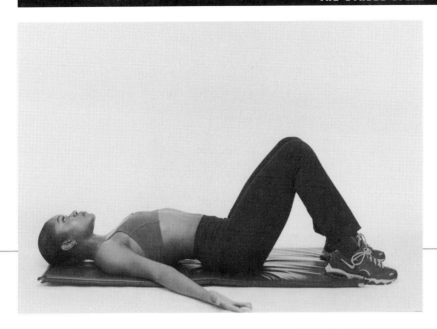

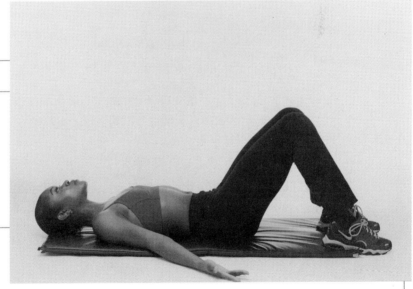

Lying pelvic tilt

Lie on the floor with your knees up, feet flat on the floor, arms at your sides, and palms up. Pinch your shoulder blades, flatten your lower back into the floor, and contract your abs. Do three reps, holding each rep for five seconds. Remember to breathe out during the contraction phase.

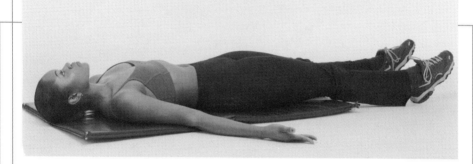

Lying pelvic tilt with legs extended

Lie on the floor with your legs fully extended. Point your toes forward while pressing your heels into the ground. Flatten the small of your lower back, trying to press it into the ground. This will help you maintain an abdominal brace. Breathe out while holding the contraction. Repeat three times, holding each rep for five seconds.

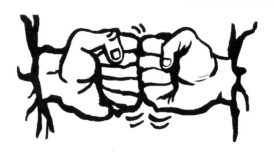

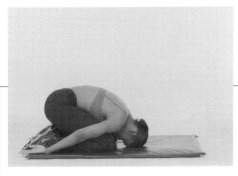

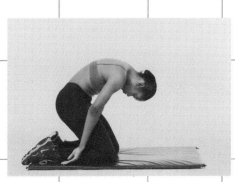

Kneeling to semi-kneeling progression

Kneel on the floor and put your forehead to the ground and your arms alongside your legs, as shown. Slowly curl up until your butt is resting on your heels and your arms are at your sides. Concentrate on maintaining the pelvic brace throughout the entire movement. Rise up to a kneeling position and extend your arms out in front of you. Hold this position for five seconds. For a greater challenge, hold 1 to 5 lb. dumbbells. Repeat three times.

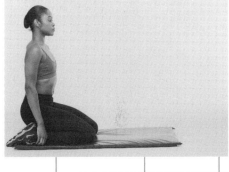

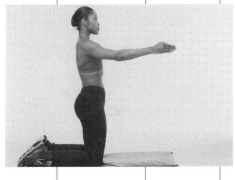

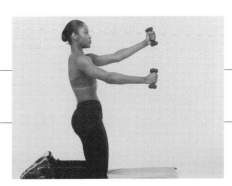

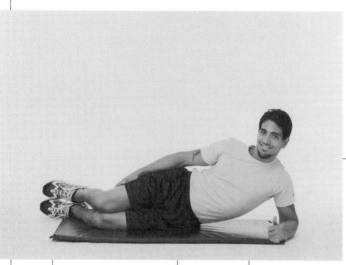

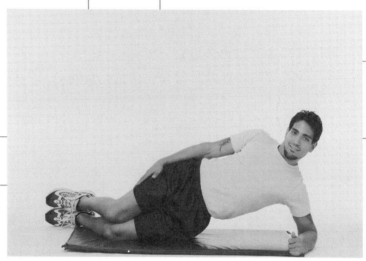

Pelvic side raises

Lie on your side with your knees bent at a 90 degree angle, so that your feet are behind you. Put one hand on your thigh and use your opposite elbow for support. Lift your hips off the ground while maintaining the abdominal brace. Exhale during lift motion. Hold five seconds. Repeat three times.

SERIES 2: BRIDGING

Bridging exercises are a more complex way of engaging your torso into a pelvic brace. Once these exercises are mastered, you abdominal, gluteal, and spinal muscular strength for the lower back greatly improves, thus assisting in stabilization during a variety of positions and activities.

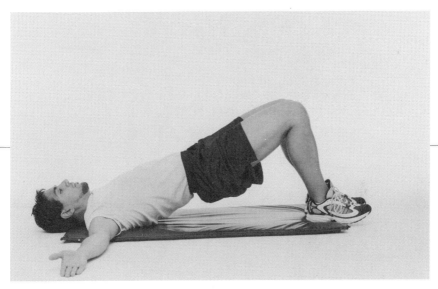

Basic bridge

Lie on your back with your knees bent, your arms extended perpendicular to your body, and your palms facing up. Lift your hips off the floor, while keeping the abdominal brace described in the previous series. Keep your hips square and do not rock side to side. Breathe out during lift and hold position for five seconds. Do three reps.

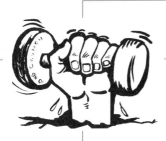

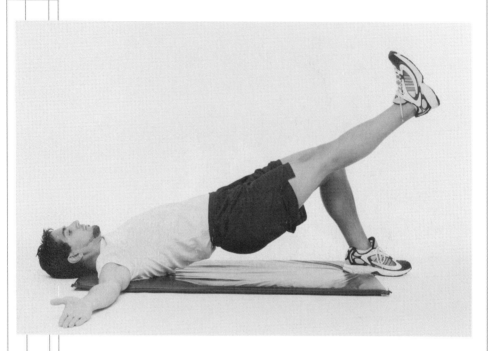

One-leg extension bridge

In the same bridge position, extend one leg so that it is in line with your body. Lead with your heel (in other words, don't point your toe). Keep your hips square during movement; do not let them rock side to side. Hold for five seconds. Lower the leg to bent knee position, then extend the opposite leg, again holding for five seconds. Lower pelvis down to the ground and repeat sequence three times. Inhale when switching legs and exhale during the opposite leg extension.

Difficulty with one-leg bridges may be due to a weak gluteus medius muscle and tight, overactive piriformis and adductors.

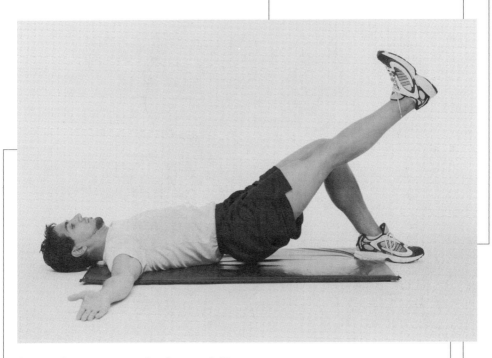

Single-leg extension bridge and dips

In the same position as the leg extension bridge, slowly dip your hips toward the floor, hold five seconds, and raise them up again. Exhale during lift phase and inhale during lowering phase. Repeat three times.

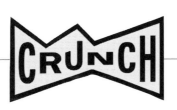

SERIES 3: PRONE RAISES

Difficulty with this progression is associated with tight psoas muscles and weak spinal erectors and traps.

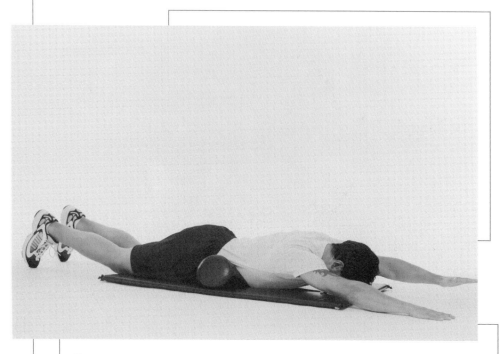

Prone arm raise

Lie on your stomach with a small pillow under your pelvis and a towel under your forehead. Your toes should touch the ground and your arms should be extended in front of you. Squeeze your shoulder blades together and raise one arm several inches off the ground while exhaling. Repeat with the other arm. Do three reps, holding each rep for five seconds.

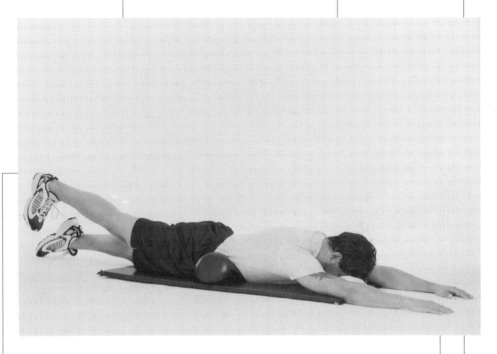

Prone leg raise

In the same prone starting position, tighten your glutes and hamstrings and raise one leg about 12 inches off the ground, keeping knee locked. Flex your foot. Repeat with the opposite leg. Do three reps, holding each for five seconds.

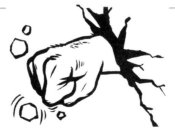

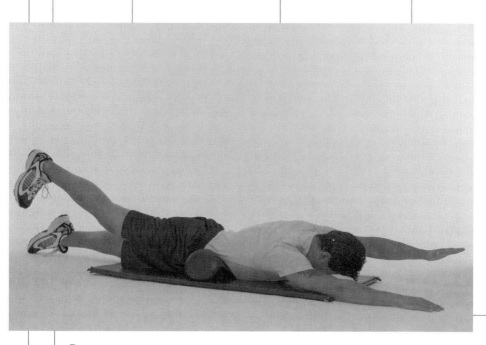

Prone crisscross

In the same prone starting position, raise your left arm and your right leg off the ground simultaneously. Hold five seconds. Repeat with the right arm and left leg. Do three reps.

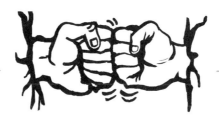

SERIES 4: QUADRIPED EXERCISES

Difficulty with these exercises is encountered when the previous prone raises are not mastered first, as well as when QLs are tight.

Do five reps of each exercise. Hold each rep for five seconds.

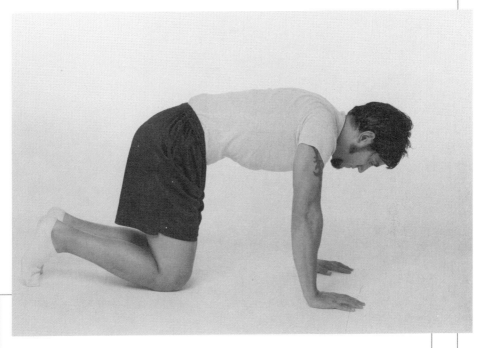

The Quadriped

Get on all fours on the floor and face down. Do a posterior pelvic tilt while pinching your shoulder blades together.

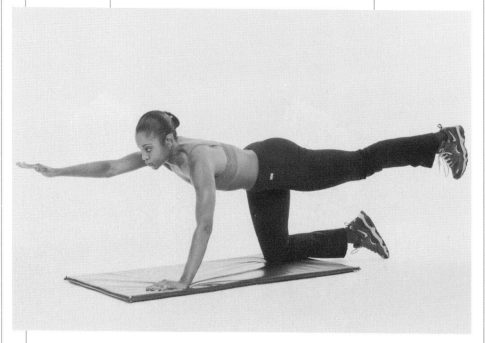

Quadriped crisscross

Get down on the floor on all fours. Look down at the floor and keep a slight, natural (i.e., unpronounced) arch in your back. Raise your right arm in front of you so that it is in line with your torso, while extending your left leg behind you so that it is also in line with your torso. Repeat with the left arm and right leg. Maintain pelvic brace throughout exercise as to prevent loss of balance and swaying side to side. Do five reps, holding each rep for five seconds.

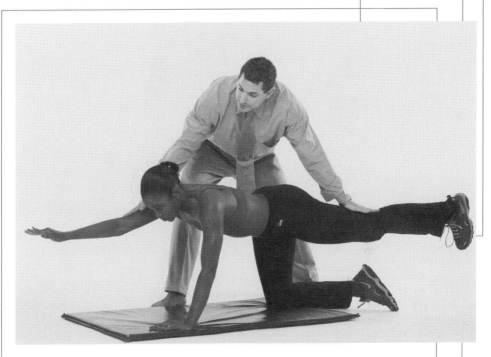

Quadriped crisscross with resistance

Perform the same exercise with resistance by having someone press down gently on your extended arm and leg. Again, try to maintain balance and pelvic brace.

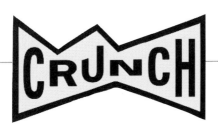

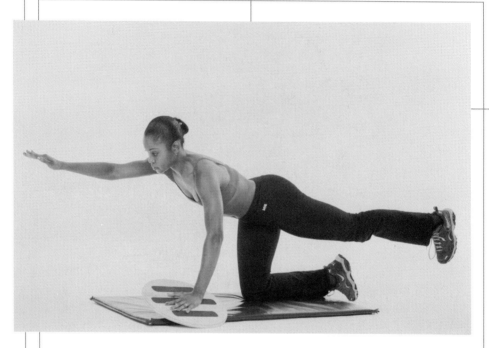

Optional: Quadriped rotation on balance board

Perform the quadriped crisscross with one hand resting on a balance board. (Extremely difficult.)

SERIES 5: TRUNK CURLS

Difficulty with these exercises is encountered when spinal erectors and hip flexors are too tight and overactive. Neck pain during the exercise can also indicate cervical spine dysfunction (requiring chiropractic care). Do three sets of 20 reps.

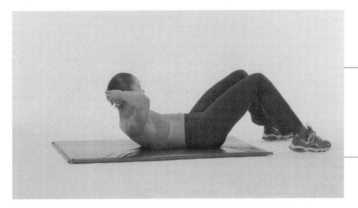

Trunk curls

Lie on the floor in the sit-up position, knees bent, feet flat on the floor, and hands behind your head. While maintaining a pelvic tilt, raise your shoulders toward your knees, then slowly lower your upper body to the floor. If your feet rise from the floor, then you're trying to crunch up too high. Do *not* anchor your legs or have someone hold them down as this will target your hip flexors and potentially injure your lower back.

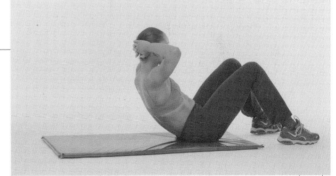

Reverse trunk curl

Start in the position shown and slowly lower your body (taking five seconds) till your shoulder blades touch the floor. Do *not* sit up to this position—push up to it with your hands.

SERIES 6: MIDDLE BACK STABILIZATION 1

Do three reps of each exercise. Hold each rep for five seconds. Use up to 5 lbs. for each exercise.

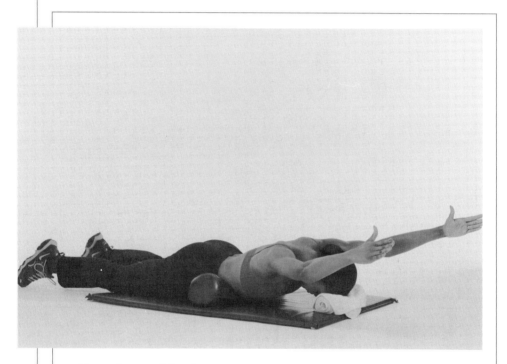

Prone forward flexion

Lie on your stomach with a small pillow under your pelvis and a towel under your forehead. Pinch your shoulder blades together and raise your arms in front of your head, as shown. Exhale during lift phase.

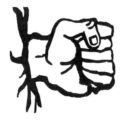 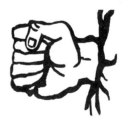

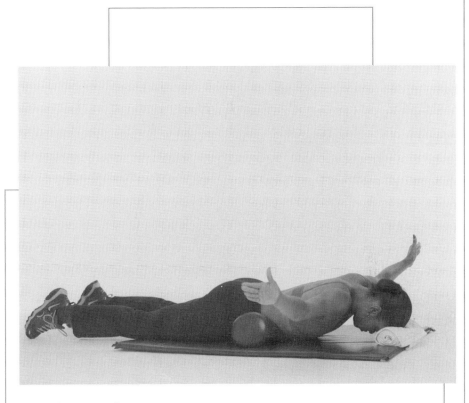

Prone horizontal retraction

In the same prone position, pinch your shoulder blades together and raise your arms out to your sides as shown. Exhale during lift phase.

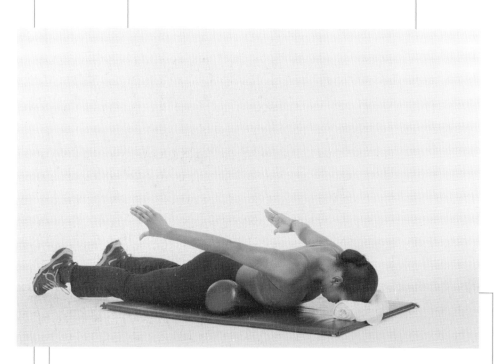

Prone rear extension

In the same prone position, pinch your shoulder blades together and extend your arms behind you, as shown. Exhale during lift phase.

SERIES 7: LUNGES AND SQUATS

Difficulty with lunges occurs when hip flexors of the rear leg and hamstrings of the front leg are too tight and when ankle or knee weakness exists.

Do three sets of 10 reps for each exercise.

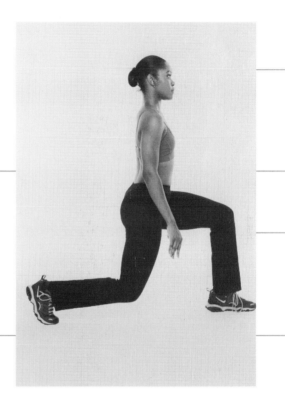

Lunges

Lunge forward, bringing your back knee to the ground while maintaining a pelvic brace. Make sure your front knee does not go beyond your front toes. Rise back up by squeezing glutes and keeping torso upright. Repeat with the opposite leg. Once you've completed three sets of 10 reps lunging forward, do another three sets lunging backwards.

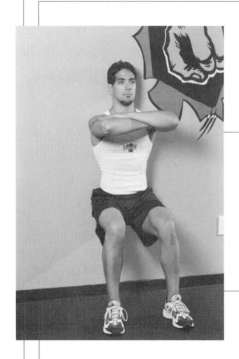

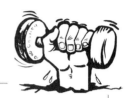

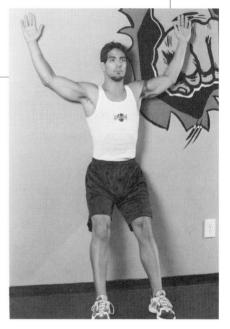

Wall squats

Stand with your back against a wall and your feet about a foot and a half away from it. Cross your arms in front of you and squat down. Try to keep your low back flat against the wall. As you rise back up, squeeze your glutes, slightly arch your low back, and extend your arms over your head. Try to keep your arms flat against the wall, but do not let your lower back sway (i.e., keep a pelvic brace throughout the movement).

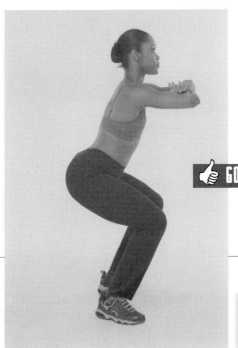

GOOD FORM

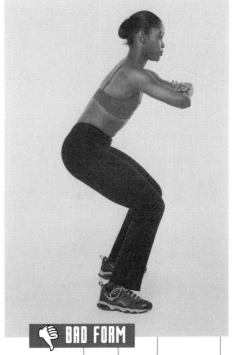

BAD FORM

Free squats

With your feet shoulder width apart and slightly turned out, and your arms crossed in front of you, squat down as low as you can until your legs almost form a 90 degree angle at the knees. Maintain a natural curve to your spine—do not attempt to flatten or round your back as in the second photo; doing so may cause you to "throw your back out" and possibly cause serious injury to your lumbar spinal disks. Squeeze your glutes and hamstrings and raise yourself up to the starting position.

Difficulty with free squats occurs when adductors are too tight and gluteus maximus and spinal erectors are weak.

SERIES 8: PHYSIOBALL PELVIC STABILIZATION

Physioball exercises are more difficult than the previous floor exercises. Do not move on to these exercises until you have mastered the previous ones. Do five reps of each exercise. Hold each rep for five seconds.

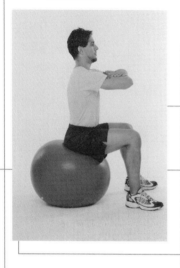

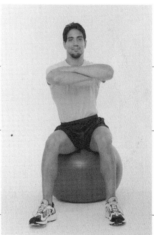

Pelvic tilts

With your arms crossed in front of you, sit on the physioball. Gently bounce, then rock your pelvis from side to side and from front to back. Find neutral spine position, i.e., a position that feels comfortable and stress-free to your spine. Then brace your abs and hold the position for five seconds.

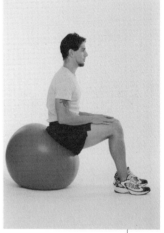

This series of exercises is intended as a warm-up to loosen your spine.

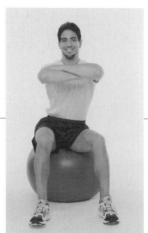

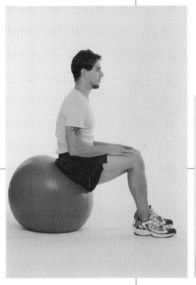

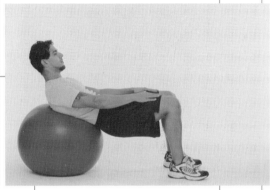

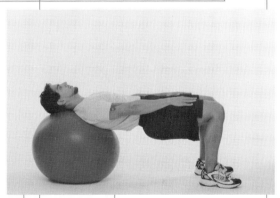

Sit-to-bridge

Sitting on the ball in neutral spine position, slowly roll back so that the ball is resting under your shoulder blades and supporting your neck. This is the bridge position. Breathe out while going into the bridge, then hold the position for five seconds. Breathe in while going back into the seated position. Repeat three times.

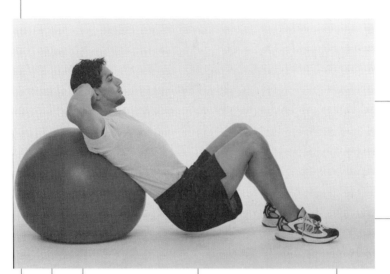

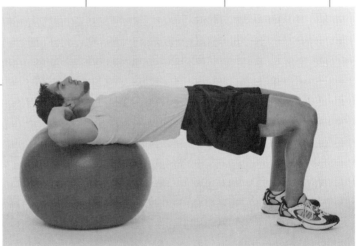

Bridge-ups

Sit on the floor with your shoulder blades resting on the ball, your hands behind your head, and your knees bent. Slowly raise your hips until you are in the bridge position. Maintain a posterior pelvic tilt throughout the entire movement. Breathe out during lift phase; breathe in while lowering.

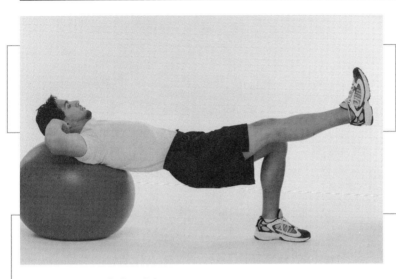

Bridge-ups with leg lifts

In the bridge position, with your hands behind your head, fully extend one leg (leading with your heel, not your toe). Hold for five seconds. Repeat with the opposite leg.

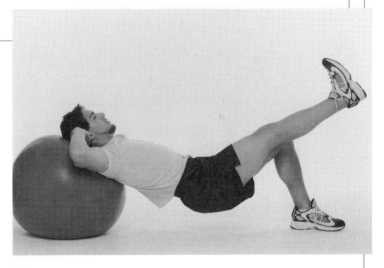

One-leg bridge dips

Perform the bridge with one leg extended, then slowly lower your hips toward the ground. Hold dip for five seconds. Rise up and repeat with the opposite leg. Do three reps.

SERIES 9: AB STABILIZATION

Do three sets of 20 reps each.

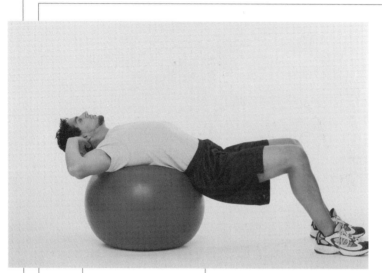

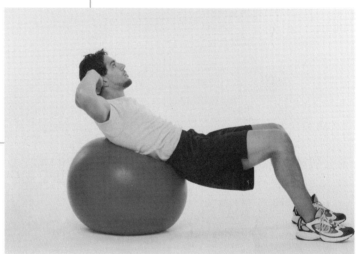

Lower trunk curl

Lie with the ball under your upper back, your hands behind your head, your knees bent, and your feet flat on the floor. Curl up slightly. Remember to keep your glutes and hamstrings activated during the entire movement to assist in pelvic bracing. This curl targets your upper abs.

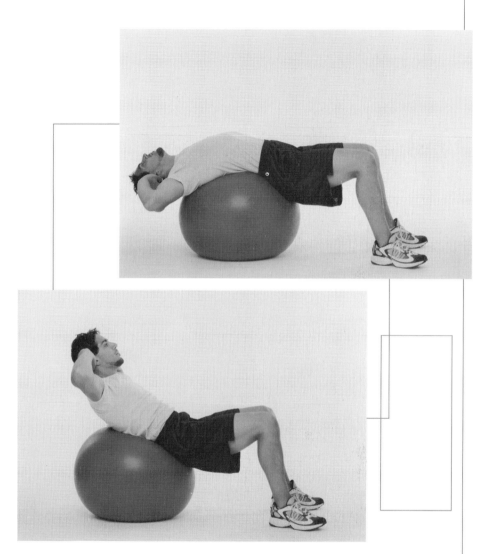

High trunk curl

Repeat the previous exercise, only this time, start with the ball under your lower back. This curl targets your lower abs.

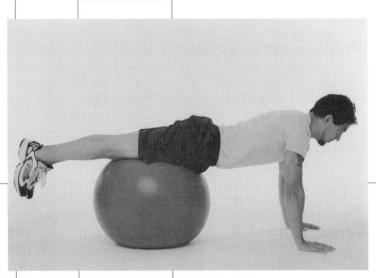

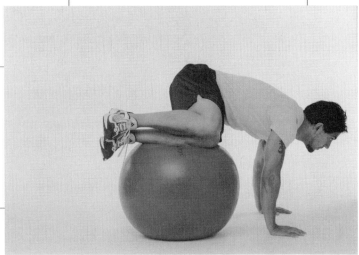

Oblique skier

Face down, put your hands on the ground, and rest your thighs on the ball, as shown. Roll the ball up to your arms by moving your legs up and to the side. Repeat movement from side to side, keeping your shoulders square to the floor. This exercise targets your internal and external obliques.

SERIES 10: BACK AUTOMOBILIZATION

Automobilization exercises are designed to loosen spinal joints. They are not muscle strength or flexibility exercises.

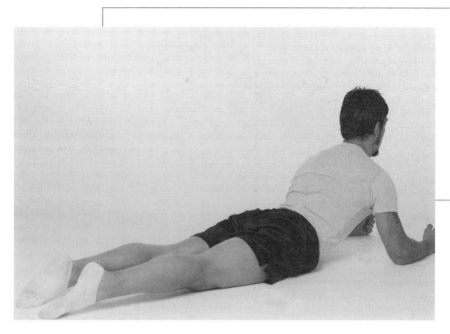

The Cobra

Lie on your stomach on the floor. Extend your upper body until you rest comfortably on your elbows. Keep your head up and your hands in fists. Hold for eight to 15 seconds. Repeat three times.

Note that it is not necessary to fully extend your spine with your arms fully locked; this will only jam the lower spine's joints and possibly lead to injury.

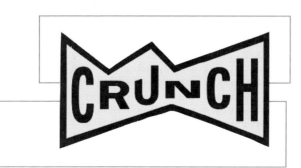

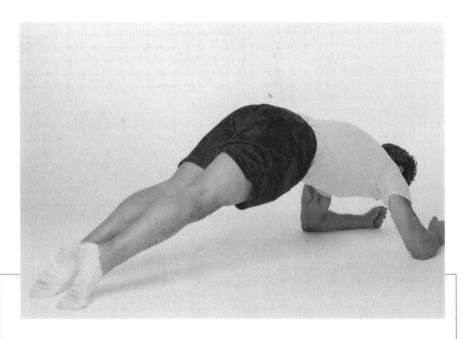

The Reverse Cobra

From the Cobra position, reverse the movement by stabilizing your abs and moving your pelvis to a posterior pelvic tilt. As you raise up, bring your hips up to a high tent position. Breathe out during reversal phase and hold for five seconds. Do three times.

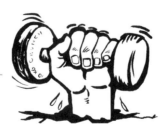

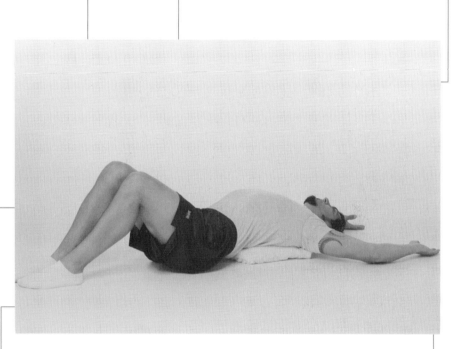

Upper back automobilization

Lie on your back on the floor. Place a folded towel, approximately 3 to 5 inches thick, between your shoulder blades, or just below. Lift your arms over your head so that your elbows nearly touch the ground and your palms face up. Do a pelvic tilt so that your lower back is almost flat. This position helps counteract a rounded upper back.

If this position is too uncomfortable, it may be a sign for you to seek the care of a chiropractor or other spinal specialist.

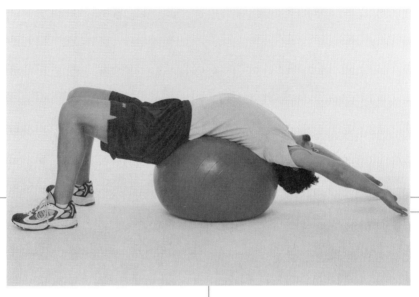

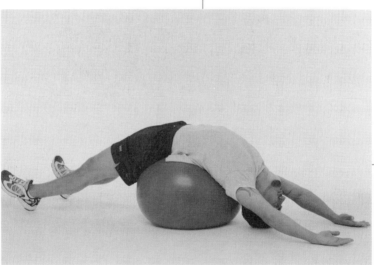

Back stretch

Lie with your back on the ball, your knees bent, and your feet flat on the floor. Slowly, extend your arms over your head, then extend your legs. Do three reps. Hold each rep for 15 to 30 seconds.

SERIES 11: MIDDLE BACK STABILIZATION 2

Do four reps of each exercise. Hold each rep for five seconds. Use up to 5 lbs. for each exercise. (Progress with weights only *after* mastering the moves without weights.)

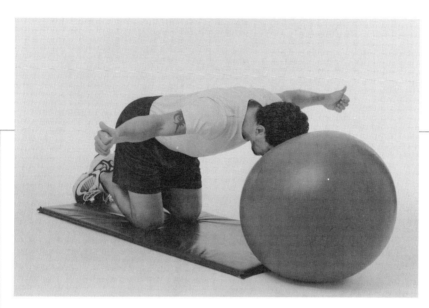

Bilateral scapular retraction—abduction

Kneel on the ground with your forehead resting on the ball. Squeeze your shoulder blades together and lift your arms as shown. Point your thumbs up. (This exercise is not advised for people with neck pain or previous neck injuries.)

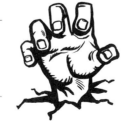

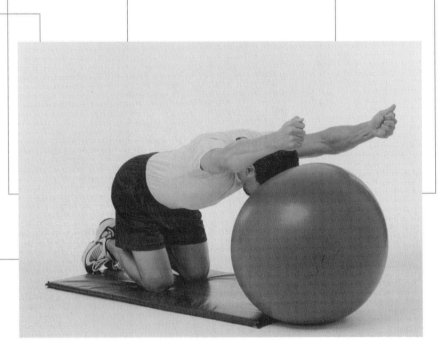

Bilateral scapular retraction—flexion

In the same position, extend your arms in front of the ball and slightly raised, as shown. Pinch your shoulder blades together and remember to keep your abs tight.

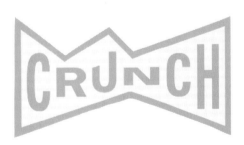

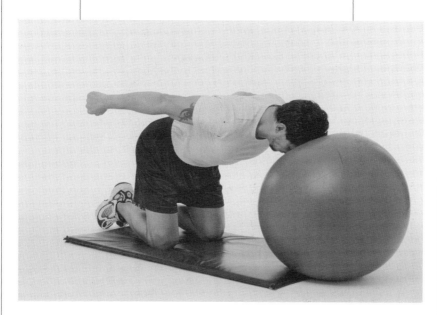

Bilateral scapular retraction—extension

In the same starting position, extend your arms behind you, as shown. Remember to squeeze your shoulder blades together.

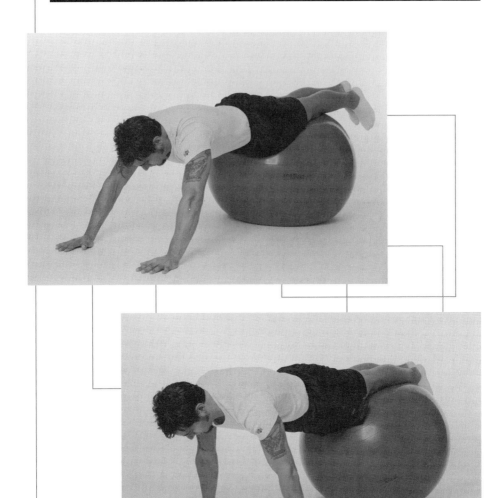

Serratus anterior protraction

Place your hands on the floor and your lower legs on the physioball, as shown. Round your shoulders and maintain this position with your elbows locked. Pull yourself forward and backward so that the ball rolls under your ankles. Maintain your pelvic brace as you roll forward and back. Do three sets of 10 reps.

This muscle is widely overlooked in most exercise programs, yet it is extremely important to proper posture.

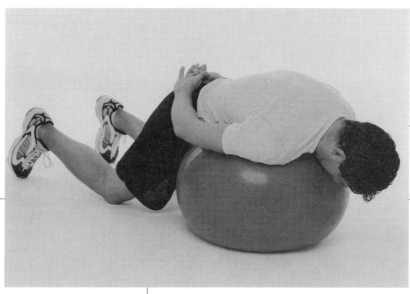

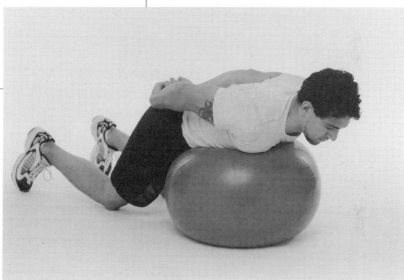

Middle back extension

Kneel and bend your torso and head over the ball. Clasp your hands behind you, at your butt. Raise your head and shoulders while pinching shoulder blades together. Try to lift your arms up while keeping your elbows locked. Do three reps. Hold each rep for five seconds.

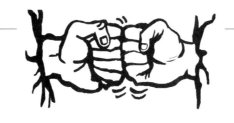

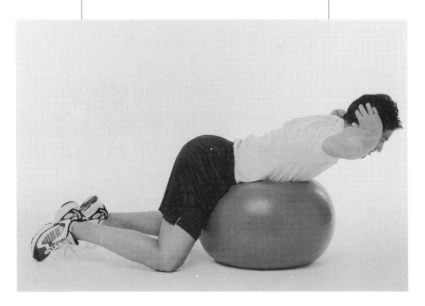

Lumbar extension

Assume the same starting position as in the previous exercise. Place your hands behind your head. Raise your shoulders and head while retracting your shoulder blades. Do three reps. Hold each rep for five seconds.

SERIES 12: SUPERMAN

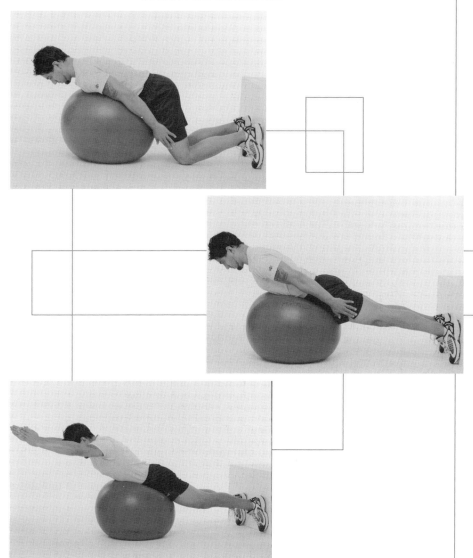

Superman

Kneel with your chest on the ball and your feet up against a wall,
shoulder width apart. Face down and maintain a neutral spine. While
keeping your arms at your sides, push off from the wall so that your
legs become fully extended and the ball rests beneath your stomach.
Pinch your shoulder blades together. Extend your arms in front of you,
palms facing each other, as shown. Hold position for five seconds. Do
five reps.

PART V
THE UPPER BODY WORKOUT

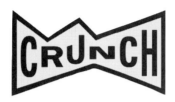

If you're able to progress through the exercises in Chapter 4, you're ready to move on to the "maintenance" exercises in Chapters 5 and 6. To keep your back muscles strong and flexible enough to promote proper posture, do the following exercise program once (or at most three times) a week. We have organized the exercise program in two parts: the upper body workout (this chapter) and the lower body workout (Chapter 6).

You can do the upper body workout one day and the lower body workout on another day, or, if you have time, you can do both workouts on the same day. But bear in mind that *you should never work the same muscle groups two days in a row*. That means you should not do the upper body workout on one day and then do it again the next day. Your muscles need time to repair and rebuild themselves after a workout. Muscles don't become stronger while you're exercising—they become stronger when you're resting *after* you've exercised. If you don't give them enough time to rest, they *will* become injured, and you *will* become weaker!

Quality vs. Quantity. A healthy back does not require more than two days a week of strengthening and stretching exercises, so don't attempt to spend hours in the gym, day after day, if you're not used to such strenuous exercise. You should concentrate on doing the exercises correctly rather than on doing more of them. Achieving the correct movement yields the most effective workout.

If you already have an exercise routine, do these posture exercises at the *end* of your workouts.

Here are some sample exercise schedules:

Monday	Upper body workout
Tuesday	Rest
Wednesday	Lower body workout
Thursday	Rest
Friday	Rest
Saturday	Upper body workout
Sunday	Rest
Monday	Lower body workout, etc.

Or:

Monday	Upper and lower body workout
Tuesday	Rest
Wednesday	Rest
Thursday	Upper and lower body workout
Friday	Rest
Saturday	Rest
Sunday	Rest

As you become stronger and the workout becomes less challenging, you can adopt the following schedule:

Monday	Upper and lower body workout
Tuesday	Rest
Wednesday	Upper and lower body workout
Thursday	Rest
Friday	Upper and lower body workout
Saturday	Rest
Sunday	Rest

Cardiovascular Exercise. A more complete exercise program would incorporate from 20 minutes to an hour of cardiovascular exercise (walking, jogging, cycling, taking an aerobics class, etc.) on two or three of the "rest" days listed above. Cardiovascular exercise works your most important muscle—your heart. It has also been clinically shown that cardiovascular exercise *relieves* lower back pain, while bed rest will actually *increase* it! (Certain cardio exercises are better for certain types of back pain, i.e., low-impact recumbant cycling may be better than high-impact aerobics depending on your condition—so consult your physician before exercising if you have back pain.)

If you add this cardio component to your schedule, always leave *one day a week for rest*—meaning no cardio or strength training exercise!

CAUTION: If you have any history of neck or back injuries or arthritis, please consult your doctor before starting this exercise program. If you have neck or back pain that does not improve after starting this exercise program, see your doctor—you could have a serious condition, such as a herniated disk or pinched nerve.

Tight Muscles to Stretch	Weak Muscles	Strengthening Exercises
levator scapulae	upper traps	shrugs
upper traps	lower traps	reverse shrugs
pectoralis major, minor	middle traps, rhomboids rear delts	partial seated rows rear delt flies
latissimus dorsi	serratus anterior	push plus
SCM, suboccipitals	deep neck flexors	chin tucks

HOW TO DO THE EXERCISES

Before stretching, do five to 10 minutes of light cardiovascular exercise, such as cycling, jogging, jumping rope, or using the UBE. This activity warms up your muscles and prevents the accumulation of lactic acid. Furthermore, it releases the buildup of pressure within synovial fluid, which lubricates your joints and helps to prevent joint and muscle injuries.

Now that you've warmed up, begin the stretches in the order presented below. Do three reps of each stretch, holding each stretch between eight and 15 seconds. Holding a stretch for longer than 15 seconds creates a rebound effect—the nerves that control the muscles perceive the muscles to be tearing (although they aren't) and counteract the stretch by tightening the muscles. Conversely, if you hold the stretch for only two to three seconds, the nerves perceive a quick, ballistic pull and, again, work to prevent the stretch by tightening the muscle.

Concentrate on breathing in while you perform each stretch. The respiratory centers of the brain assist in relaxing muscles. If you inhale while stretching, you will enhance the effectiveness of the stretch by utilizing the respiratory center of your brain to relax the muscle. Conversely, if you exhale during the stretch, you actually work against your goal and may tighten the muscle you're trying to relax.

Proceed then to the strengthening exercises. For each strengthening exercise, complete one set of 15 repetitions. Rest for 30 seconds between exercises. When you can do the entire workout without too much effort, work your way up to performing three "supersets" of the entire workout, taking a minimal amount of time between exercises. This means you would go through the workout once, performing one set of 15 reps for each exercise, then repeat the entire workout twice more. Cool down with five to 10 minutes of cardio exercise. (If you don't have machines at your disposal, see Series 6 and 11 in Chapter 4.)

Remember: Stabilize your spine in a neutral position and maintain a pelvic brace, as described in Chapter 4, before starting each exercise!

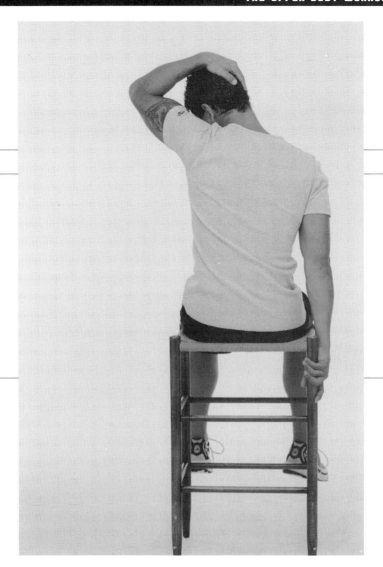

Levator scapula stretch

Sit on a bench or stool and place your left hand over the back right side of your head. Use your right hand to hold onto the chair or simply place it behind your lower back, palm facing up. Gently pull your head down and rotate your chin to the left. Repeat on the opposite side.

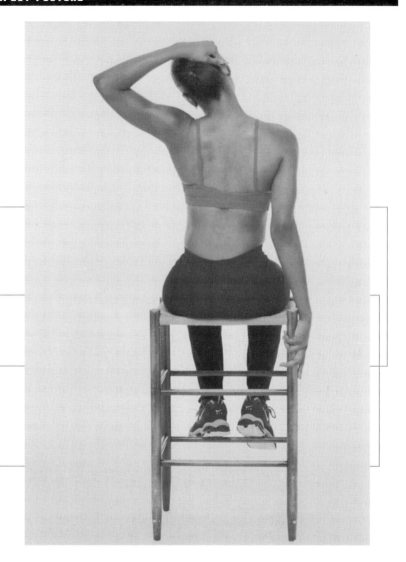

Upper trap stretch

Perform the same stretch as the previous one, only gently pull your head to the side. Do not rotate chin or turn head.

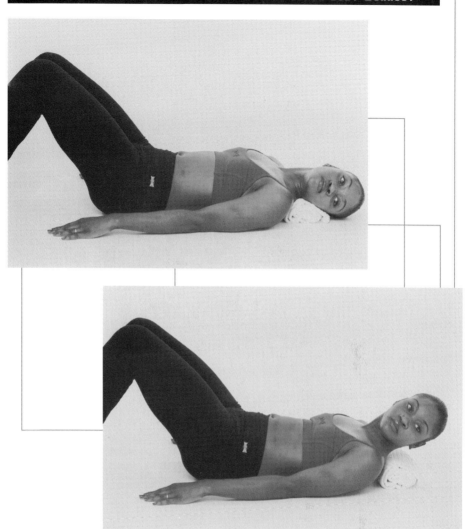

SCM stretch

Lie on the floor with your knees bent, your feet flat on the floor, and your arms at your sides. If uncomfortable, you can put a rolled-up towel under your neck. Face left, inhale, and raise your head off the floor a few inches. Hold for three to five seconds. Exhale and place your head back down. Repeat, facing the opposite direction. (If your neck hurts or if you become lightheaded, consult your physician—do not try to "push through the pain.")

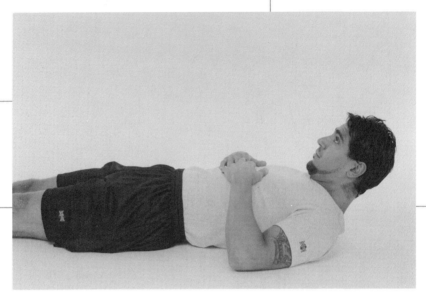

Suboccipitals stretch

Lie on the floor with your legs fully extended and your hands clasped over your chest. With your head facing up, breathe in and lift your head off the floor, tucking your chin to your chest.

STRONG ARM TACTICS

You may want to consider doing arm exercises, such as tricep kickbacks and bicep curls, as part of your upper body workout. If you choose to work out these muscles, do them first—*before* you've done the back exercises. *Note:* Overdevelopment of biceps may round shoulders forward and actually contribute to poor posture, as well as eventually leading to rotator cuff injuries. Oftentimes, people focus on developing strong arm and upper back muscles, building muscle on top of poor posture, which complicates their posture problems and increases their risk of injury.

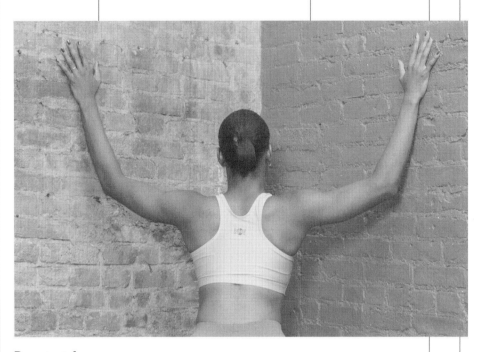

Pec stretch

Stand about a foot away from a corner and place your hands on the walls, slightly above your head. Keep your head facing forward and tilted slightly up. Keeping bent elbows, breathe in as you lean into the corner. Breathe out as you push yourself out of the corner.

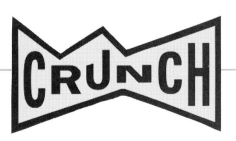

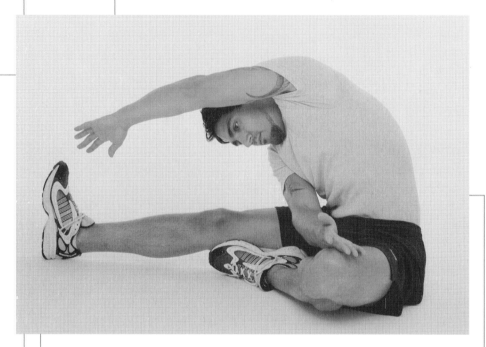

Lat stretch

Sit on the floor with your right leg extended out in front of you and your left leg bent out to the side. Bend forward, reaching your left arm toward your right toe. Your right arm should reach for your left knee, as shown. Repeat on the opposite side. Remember to inhale during stretch and exhale upon release.

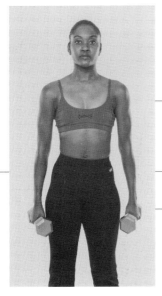
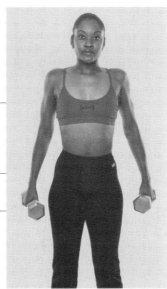

Shrugs (upper traps)

Stand straight and hold a dumbbell of comfortable weight in each hand at hip level. Pinch your shoulder blades together. Lift your shoulders, as if to touch your ears. Maintain a neutral pelvis throughout the movement. Do not roll shoulders forward and backward as this may cause premature arthritic stress to your joints.

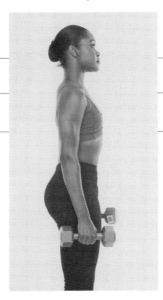
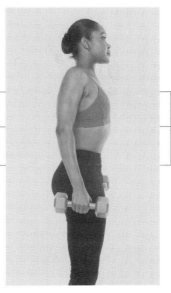

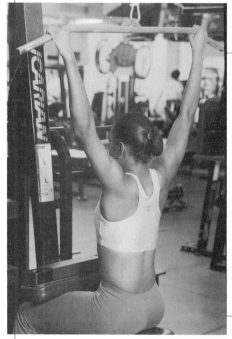

Reverse shrugs (lower traps)

Sit at the lat pull-down machine and find your neutral
spinal position. Contract
your abs to maintain a stable
spine as you pull down the
weight slightly by "shrug-
ging" your shoulders down.

Do not bend your elbows.
This exercise uses your lower
traps and is performed by
lowering your shoulder
blades only. Remember not
to flex your head down. Look
straight ahead to prevent
rounding of the neck and
upper back.

The more common exer-
cise using this equipment is

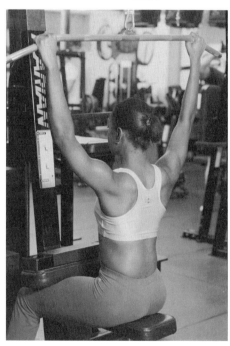

the lat pull-down, which, by training your lats, contributes to the
rounded upper back and shoulder postures, which in turn can lead
to back injuries.

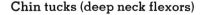

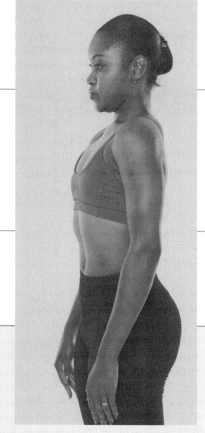

Chin tucks (deep neck flexors)

Stand up straight with your arms at your sides. Retract your jaw—think about trying to give yourself double—or triple—chins. Keep your head up.

LET SOMEONE ELSE WORK YOUR MUSCLES

For optimum back health, consider getting a massage once a month. Massage helps to stimulate blood flow to muscles, loosen tight muscles, relieve tension, and promote relaxation. It also helps to eliminate lactic acid, a chemical waste product that builds up in muscle tissue during exercise.

Swedish massage is the most popular form of massage therapy. The therapist manipulates muscles lightly or deeply, depending on your comfort level.

While Swedish massage focuses on muscle manipulation, Shiatsu massage is energy oriented. The therapist locates and stimulates specific energy pressure points on the body. This increase of energy flow in the body assists the functioning of internal organs.

Reflexology focuses on loosening joints in the hands and feet to clear blockages along the energy meridians that lead to the body's vital organs.

Finally, for a complete assessment of your back health, consider visiting a doctor of chiropractic. Even healthy backs can benefit from a chiropractor's manipulation once a month, as this will stimulate your entire neuromusculoskeleton, thus promoting the spine's longevity by helping to prevent degenerative arthritis and osteoporosis as you age.

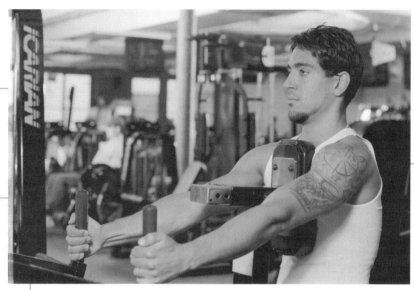

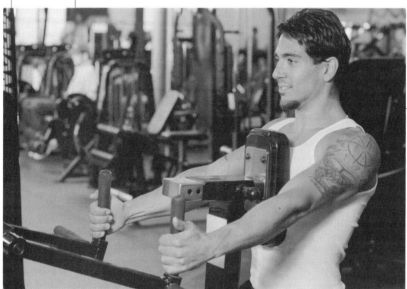

Partial seated rows (middle traps)

Sit at the seated row machine so that your chest is against the pad, your hands grip the handles, and your back is in neutral spine position. Squeeze your shoulder blades together to bring the weight back. *Do not* yank the handles back by bending your elbows—that movement does not work the intended muscles.

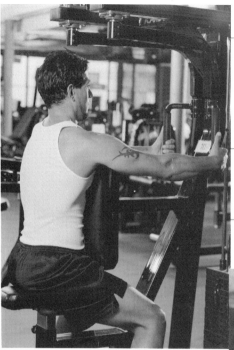

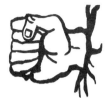

Rear delt flies

Sit at the rear delt machine with your chest against the pad and your back in a stable, neutral spine position. Bring the weights out to the side by squeezing your shoulder blades together.

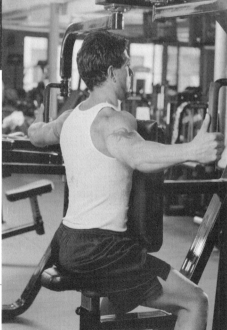

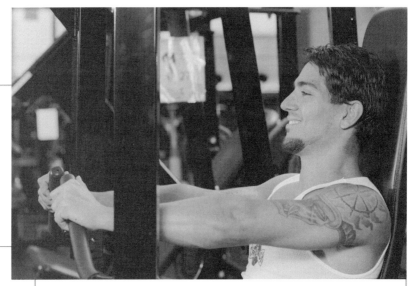

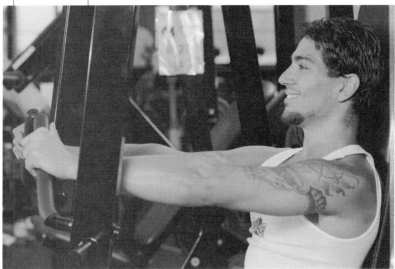

Push plus (serratus anterior)

Sit on the chest press machine with your hands gripping the handles. Find your neutral spine position. Push forward to lock your elbows. Contract your abs and maintain a stable pelvis. Squeeze your shoulder blades together to start, then round your shoulders forward by separating your shoulder blades to finish. Do not bend your elbows, as this will not work the intended muscles.

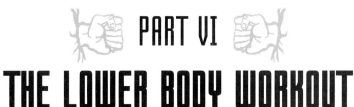

PART VI
THE LOWER BODY WORKOUT

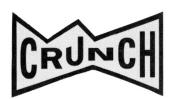

This workout helps prevent the Lower Crossed Syndrome, which was described in Chapter 3. As with the upper body workout, you should not attempt this workout until you have mastered the floor stabilization exercises in Chapter 4.

Following the schedule you chose in Chapter 5, incorporate the following lower body workout into your exercise program. As you did before the upper body workout, begin with a five- to 10-minute cardio warm-up. Then, hold each stretch between eight and 15 seconds. Perform each stretch three times. For each strengthening exercise, complete one set of 15 repetitions. Work yourself up to performing three supersets of the entire workout. And remember to stabilize your spine before each exercise!

Tight Muscles to Stretch	Weak Muscles	Strengthening Exercise
psoas, rectus femoris	gluteus maximus	crunches (various)
spinal erectors	abdominals	cable kickbacks
hamstrings	spinal erectors	reverse hyperextensions
adductors, QLs, piriformis, TFL	gluteus medius	cable kickouts
	quadriceps	wall squats

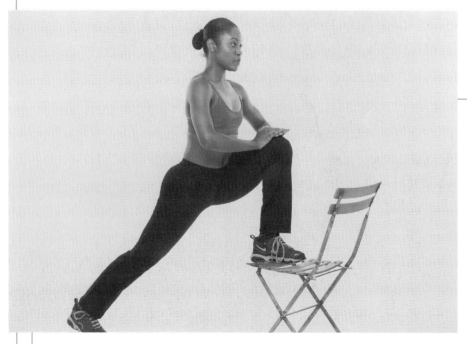

Psoas stretch

Lunge onto a chair. Maintain a pelvic tilt by contracting your abs. Press your back heel to the floor. Squeeze your glutes. You should feel the stretch in front of your thigh and into your groin. Rotate your rear foot inward to keep it in a straight line with your thigh. Do *not* rotate your back foot out. Repeat with the opposite leg.

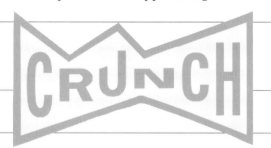

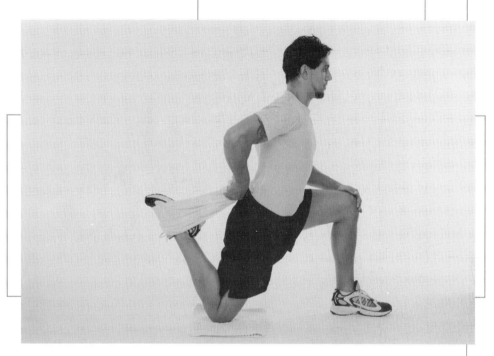

Rectus femoris stretch

Lunge onto the floor and bring your back knee all the way to the floor. Wrap a towel around your back foot and pull it gently toward your torso. Lunge forward to accentuate the stretch. Remember to keep your torso upright—do not lean forward as this lessens the effectiveness of the stretch. Repeat with the opposite leg.

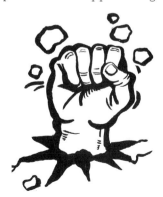

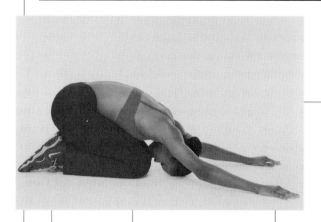

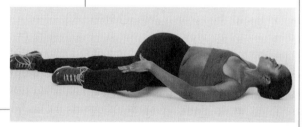

Spinal erectors stretches

1. Kneel on the floor so that your butt rests on your heels, your back is rounded, your forehead touches the ground, and your arms are extended in front of you. Breathe in and reach forward with your arms while keeping your butt on your heels.

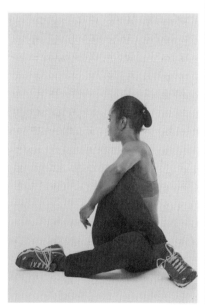

2. Lie on the floor with your legs extended. While facing up, cross your right leg over your left leg, bending your right knee up to hip level. The bent knee should touch the floor. Repeat on the opposite side. Try to keep both shoulders square on the floor and breathe in during the stretch.

3. Sit on the floor with your left leg bent out to the side, trying to touch the floor. Bend your right knee up and cross your right leg over your left thigh, as shown. Turn your body to face right. Breathe in during the stretch. Repeat on the opposite side.

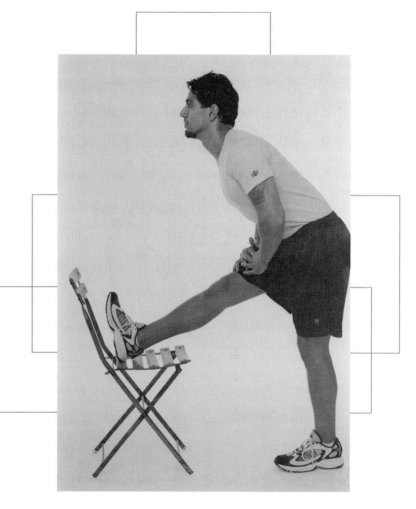

Hamstring stretch

Stand and place one heel on a chair. Keeping your back slightly arched, fold forward at your pelvis and lean into your leg. *Don't round your back to try to bring your chin to your knee.* Keep elevated knee straight,toes pointed toward forehead and keep a slight bend in the standing knee. Repeat with the opposite leg.

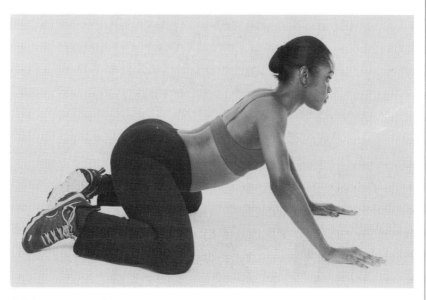

Adductor stretch

Get down on the floor on all fours. Slowly spread your knees out to the sides, and thrust chest toward the floor.

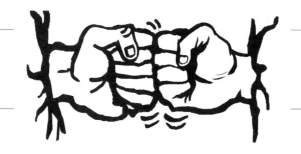

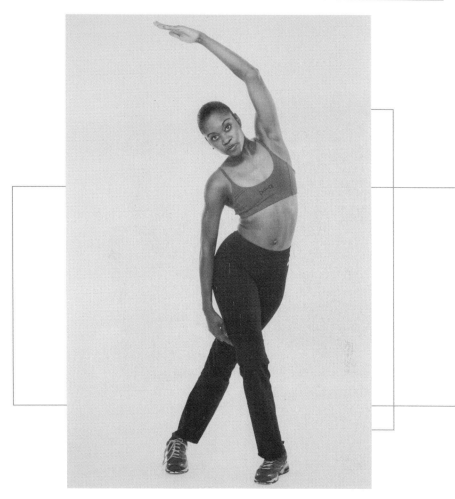

QL stretch

Stand up straight with your legs together. With your left leg, take a step back and to the right so that your left leg crosses behind your right leg, as shown. Reach your left arm over your head and bend to the right. Breathe in as you stretch and reach up toward the ceiling. Repeat on the opposite side. Tight QLs are the most common culprit behind low back pain.

TFL stretch

Take the same position as above, only sit slightly into it, i.e., flex your upper body foward slightly.

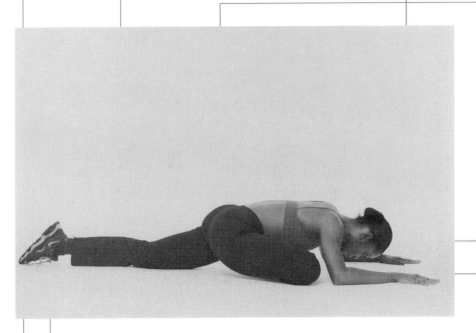

Piriformis stretch

Lie on your stomach on your right shin with your left leg fully extended behind you, and face down. Your right knee should be bent near chest level. Try to bring your right foot toward your left shoulder. Repeat with the opposite leg.

When tight, the piriformis commonly causes sciatica (pain and numbness that radiates down the back , part of the buttock, hamstring, and into the calves and feet).

Glute medius stretch

Sit on a chair and cross one ankle on your opposite knee. Lean forward, reaching your arms in front of your knees, as if you're trying to touch the floor.

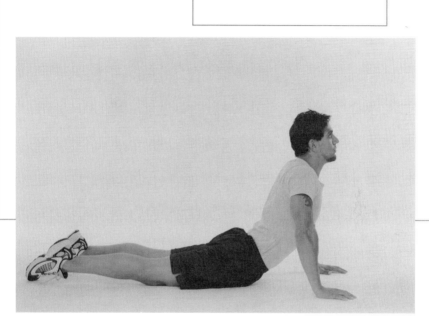

Lumbar extension

Lie on your stomach on the floor. Push your shoulders up, extending your arms and facing up, as shown. If this position is too difficult, then bend your elbows and lean on your forearms.

ABS

Do three sets of 20 reps for each of the following exercises.

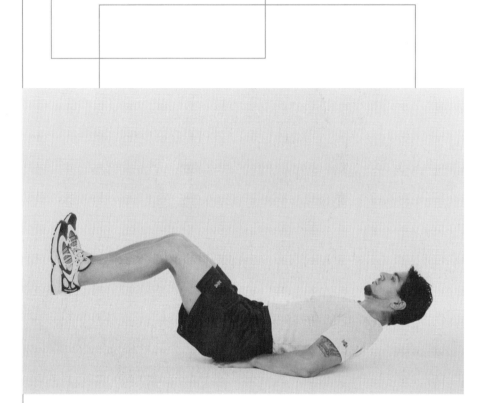

Legs lifts (lower abs)

Lie on your back on the floor and put your hands under your butt. Maintaining a flat lower back, lift your legs off the ground 10 to 12 inches, bend your knees, and lift your head, as shown. Now, slowly lower your ankles until they're slightly off the ground and reverse action back up again. Remember to maintain a flat back throughout the movement, as a swayed spine may strain the lower back.

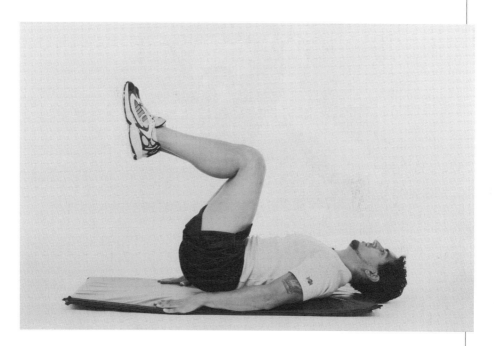

Hip thrust (lower abs)

Lie on your back on the floor and put your arms at your sides. Lift your legs and bend your knees, as shown. Raise your hips slightly off the floor (2 to 3 inches). Do not bring your knees toward your head—simply lift them straight up and down.

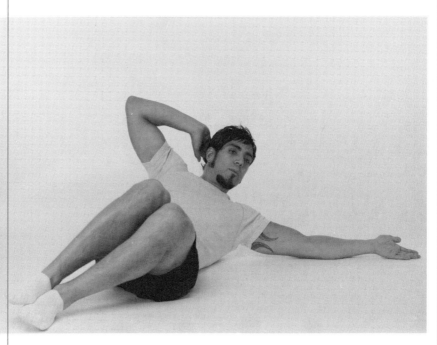

Internal oblique crunch

Lie on the floor with left arm straight out to the side and the right arm bent at the elbow so that its hand comes to your right ear. Bend your knees slightly and rotate them to the left, keeping your ankles on the floor. Crunch obliquely to your left side, raising your right shoulder toward your knees. Repeat on the opposite side.

Internal obliques are commonly overlooked, yet they are crucial for the full development of lower back stabilization.

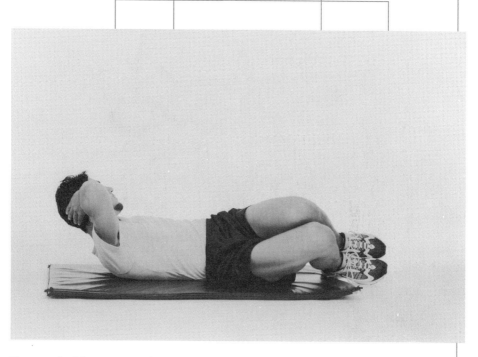

External oblique crunch

Assume the same position as you did for the previous crunch, only rotate your legs to the opposite side and crunch your torso away from your legs.

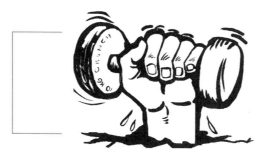

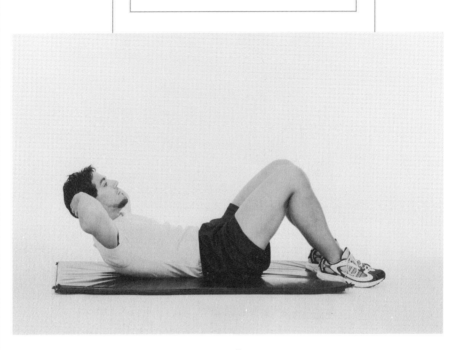

Standard crunch (transverse abs)

Lie on your back on the floor with your hands behind your head, your knees bent, and your feet flat on the floor. Crunch up slightly, bringing your shoulder blades approximately 8 to 10 inches off the ground between reps. Do not let your shoulders touch the ground between reps.

If your neck is weak or juts forward, try crossing your arms in front of your chest as this will lessen the load and make the exercise easier.

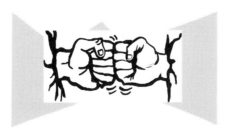

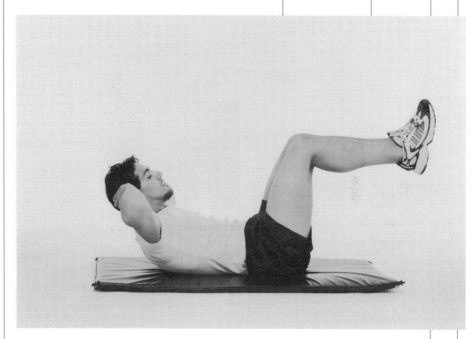

Complete crunch (upper abs)

Take the same starting position as the previous crunch, only bring your feet off the ground so that your shins are perpendicular to your thighs, as shown. Crunch up as before, remembering to keep your hips and knees locked, using only your torso during the exercise. Do not bring your knees toward your chest as this will train your hip flexors and eventually injure your lower back.

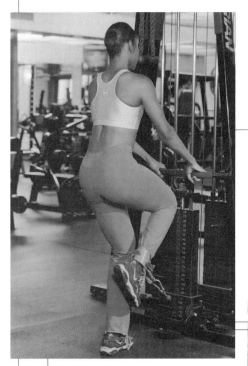

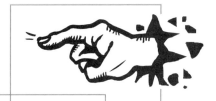

Cable kickbacks (glute max)

Face the weight machine and attach the ankle belt around one ankle. Hold the bar for support. Maintaining a stable, neutral spine, bring one knee up, then kick back so that your back leg is fully extended. Keep a slight bend in the opposite knee. Keep your hips square and face forward—do not twist your pelvis as this will create torsion and place undue stress on your lower back. Repeat with the other leg.

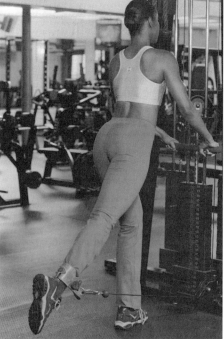

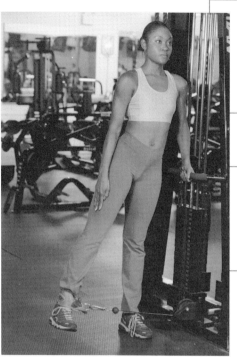

Cable kickouts (glute medius)

With the ankle belt around one ankle and the opposite hand on the handle for support, kick out to the side slightly. *Do not kick out high, as in the second photo.* This overtrains the QL and will lead to low back injuries. Repeat with the opposite leg.

BAD FORM

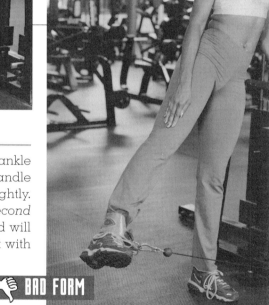

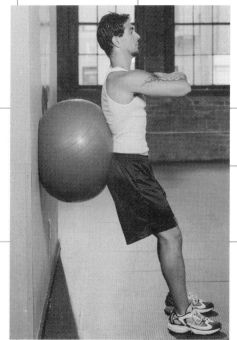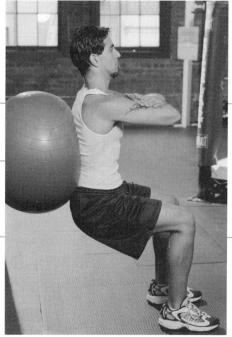

Physioball wall squats (hams, glutes, quads, and lumbar erectors)

Place the physioball between a wall and the small of your back. With your arms crossed in front of you, squat down and rise back up again. The ball helps cushion the lower back and prevents swayback during squats.

A LEG UP

To complete your lower body workout, you may want to consider doing leg exercises, such as leg presses, leg extensions, leg curls, inner and outer thigh presses, and calf raises. If you choose to work these muscles, do them first—*before* you've done the back exercises.

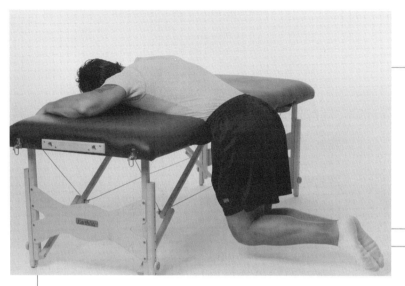

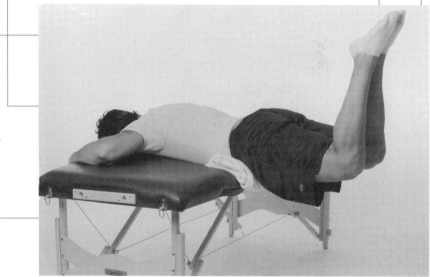

Reverse hyperextensions (lumbar erectors)

Lie on your stomach on a bench with your hips resting on the edge of the bench and your knees bent, as shown. If you have a pronounced low back sway, then roll up a towel and place it under your pelvis to reduce the sway. Lift your feet so that your thighs become parallel to the floor. This is the most intense exercise in the sequence. If you are unable to perform this exercise comfortably, return to Chapter 4 and work on strengthening your lower back muscles.

EXERCISES TO AVOID

In short, the four scenarios below are the most common exercise errors made in the health club setting.

1. Do not do hyperextensions. In this popular gym exercise, the unwitting person lies, from the hips down, on an inclined bench or roman chair. She locks her legs in place by placing her ankles under roller pads. Her hands are clasped behind her head. She leans down, then raises herself back up.

This exercise causes joint compression, leading to nerve damage. It also causes premature arthritis and can lead to eventual disk injuries.

The better exercise is the reverse hyperextension, described in this workout.

2. Do not do side-to-side dumbbell lifts. Bending your torso from side to side while holding dumbbells trains your QLs, not your abdominal obliques. Your QLs are easily overdeveloped, so doing a specific exercise for them merely increases the force on your lower spine (and increases the risk of disk herniations). Some athletes, such as hockey and baseball players and discus and javelin throwers, need to train their QLs to accommodate their sport, but most people should avoid this exercise.

3. Avoid flexing your neck when performing exercises not intended for your neck. For example, many people flex their necks forward while doing the leg press. This can sprain your neck and put pressure on your lower back by straining the spinal canal and spinal cord.

4. Avoid ab exercises that anchor your ankles in place. Abdominal muscles can lift your torso only about 30 degrees, which should just bring your shoulder blades off the ground. When you perform ab exercises that bring your torso higher, you begin to activate your hip flexor muscles. By anchoring your ankles (underneath a roller bar, for example) you primarily use your hip flexor muscles to perform the movement—providing no benefit to your abs. These hip flexors are attached to the front part of the lumbar spine, and if they become overdeveloped, the hip flexors tug the spine forward, thus increasing the curve in the lower back and causing compression of the spinal joints. The overuse of these muscles is most often responsible for common sprains and strains to the spine (as in "throwing your back out"), which ultimately result in disk injuries and arthritis. In short, the best place to do ab exercises is the floor.

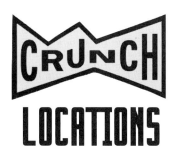

LOCATIONS

Where to work out, pretend to work out, or just stand around calling our personal trainers "Hans" and "Franz" under your breath.

NEW YORK CITY

404 Lafayette Street
(Astor Place and 4th Avenue)
212.614.0120

54 East 13th Street
(University and Broadway)
212.475.2018

162 West 83rd Street
(Columbus and Amsterdam)
212.875.1902

623 Broadway (at Houston)
212.420.0507

152 Christopher Street
(at Greenwich Street)
212.366.3725

1109 Second Avenue
(at 59th Street)
212.758.3434

144 W. 38th St.
(7th Ave. & Broadway)
212.869.7788

LOS ANGELES

8000 Sunset Blvd.
(West Hollywood)
323.654.4550

SAN FRANCISCO

1000 Van Ness Avenue
(Geary and O'Farrell)
415.931.1100

MISSION VIEJO

The Kaleidoscope Center
27741 Crown Valley Parkway
949.582.8181

MIAMI

1259 Washington Avenue
(South Beach)
305.674.8222

ATLANTA AREA
[ALL LOCATIONS: 800.660.5433]

Crunch Club Cobb
North by NW Office Park
1775 Water Place
Atlanta, GA 30339

Crunch Gwinnett
Gwinnett Prado
2300 Pleasant Hill Road
Duluth, GA 30136

Crunch Town Center
Main Street Shopping Center
2600 Prado Lane
Marietta, GA 30066

Crunch Roswell
Roswell Exchange
11060 Alpharetta Highway
Roswell, GA 30076

Crunch Buckhead
3365 Piedmont Road, Suite 1010
Atlanta, GA

Crunch Stone Mountain
Stone Mountain Square
5370 Highway 78 South
Stone Mountain, GA 30087

CHICAGO

Crunch Chicago
350 North State Street
Chicago, IL 60610
312.527.8100

TOKYO

Crunch Omotesando
4-3-24 Jingumae Sibuya

Coming soon to Las Vegas!

Visit us on the Web at
www.crunch.com

The doctor of the future will give no medicine
but will interest his patients in the care
of the human frame, in diet, and in the cause
and prevention of disease.

THOMAS EDISON

Dr. Scott G. Duke
Chiropractor

• • •

DUKE CHIROPRACTIC P.C.
270 Madison Avenue
New York, NY 10016
212.481.0066

Personal Training Coupon

15% OFF! 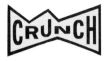 15% OFF!

IT'S EASY ... Come into any CRUNCH location and receive 15% off your first purchase of personal training. Then just sign, date, and present this coupon at the fitness desk to set up your session.

_____   _____
MEMBER NAME   SIGNATURE

_____   _____
TRAINER NAME   TRAINER SIGNATURE

_____
DATE OF SESSION

Cannot be combined with any other offer. Valid for one use only

- - - - - - - - - - - - CUT AT DOTTED LINE - - - - - - - - - - - -

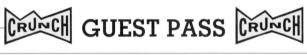

GUEST PASS

$22 value!

Must show picture ID to use facility.
The same guest may use only two guest passes per year

_____   _____
MEMBERSHIP REP   EXPIRATION DATE

OUR MISSION AND PHILOSOPHY

We at CRUNCH warmly welcome people from all walks of life,
regardless of shape, size, sex, or ability.
People don't have to be flawless to feel at home at CRUNCH. We don't care
if our members are 18 or 80, fat or thin, short or tall, muscular or mushy, blond or bald,
or anywhere in between. CRUNCH is not competitive, it is non-judgmental,
it is not elitist, it does not represent a kind of person.
CRUNCH is a gym; a movement which is growing as we continue to perfect our ability
to create an environment where our members don't feel self-conscious,
and don't worry about what others think.
At the heart of CRUNCH's core stands a tremendously experienced and energetic staff
dedicated to creating an environment where everyone feels accepted—
a truly unique place!

WWW.CRUNCH.COM

The **hottest** fitness spot on the internet!

OUR MISSION AND PHILOSOPHY

We at CRUNCH warmly welcome people from all walks of life,
regardless of shape, size, sex, or ability.
People don't have to be flawless to feel at home at CRUNCH. We don't care
if our members are 18 or 80, fat or thin, short or tall, muscular or mushy, blond or bald,
or anywhere in between. CRUNCH is not competitive, it is non-judgmental,
it is not elitist, it does not represent a kind of person.
CRUNCH is a gym; a movement which is growing as we continue to perfect our ability
to create an environment where our members don't feel self-conscious,
and don't worry about what others think.
At the heart of CRUNCH's core stands a tremendously experienced and energetic staff
dedicated to creating an environment where everyone feels accepted—
a truly unique place!

WWW.CRUNCH.COM

*The **hottest** fitness spot on the internet!*

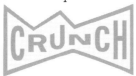

- - - - - - - - - - - CUT AT DOTTED LINE - - - - - - - - - - -

NEW YORK CITY

404 Lafayette Street
(Astor Place and 4th Street)
212.614.0120

54 East 13th Street
(University and Broadway)
212.475.2018

162 West 83rd Street
(Columbus and Amsterdam)
212.875.1902

623 Broadway (at Houston)
212.420.0507

152 Christopher Street
(at Greenwich Street)
212.366.3725

1109 Second Avenue
(at 59th Street)
212.758.3434

144 W. 38th St.
(7th Ave. & Broadway)
212.869.7788

LOS ANGELES

8000 Sunset Blvd.
(West Hollywood)
323.654.4550

SAN FRANCISCO

1000 Van Ness Avenue
(Geary and O'Farrell)
415.931.1100

MISSION VIEJO

The Kaleidoscope Center
27741 Crown Valley
  Parkway
949.582.8181

MIAMI

1259 Washington Avenue
(South Beach)
305.674.8222

ATLANTA AREA
(All locations: 800.660.5433)

Crunch Club Cobb
North by NW Office Park
1775 Water Place
Atlanta, GA 30339

Crunch Gwinnett
Gwinnett Prado
2300 Pleasant Hill Road
Duluth, GA 30136

Crunch Town Center
Main Street Shopping
  Center
2600 Prado Lane
Marietta, GA 30066

Crunch Roswell
Roswell Exchange
11060 Alpharetta Highway
Roswell, GA 30076

Crunch Buckhead
3365 Piedmont Road,
Suite 1010
Atlanta, GA

Crunch Stone Mountain
Stone Mountain Square
5370 Highway 78 South
Stone Mountain, GA 30087

CHICAGO

Crunch Chicago
350 North State Street
Chicago, IL 60610
312.527.8100

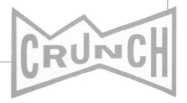

LAS VEGAS COMING SOON!